HEALING GARDENS

ROMY RAWLINGS

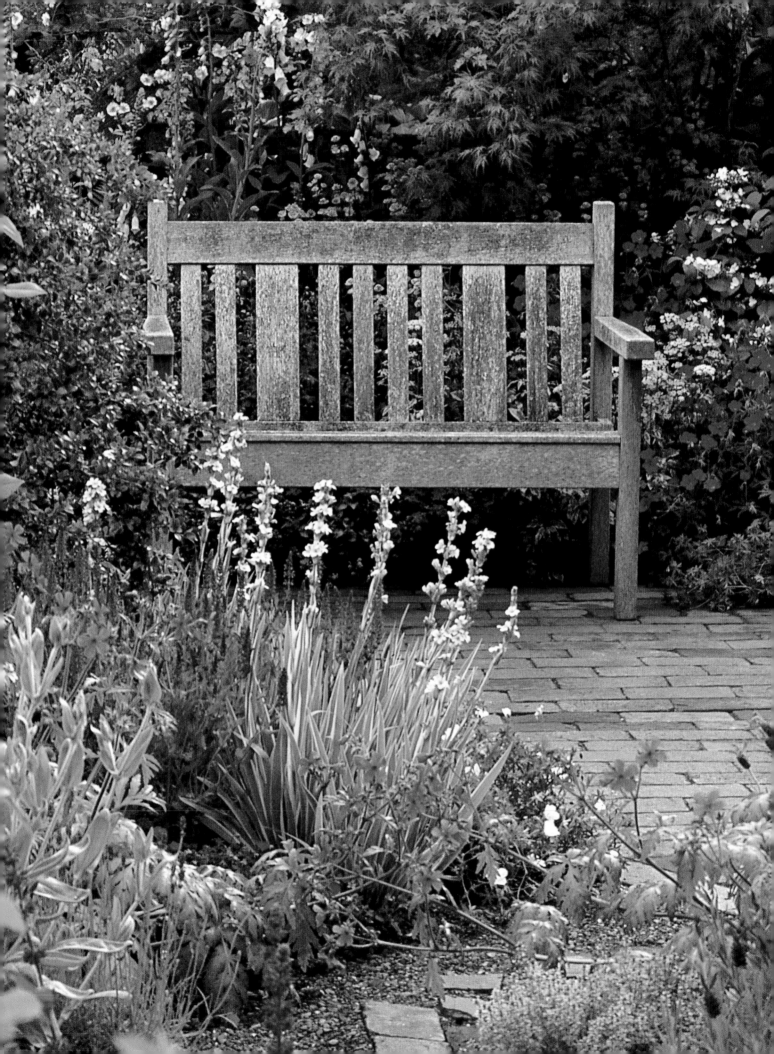

HEALING GARDENS

ROMY RAWLINGS

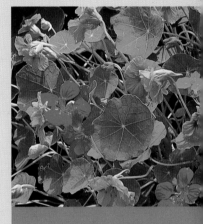

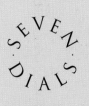

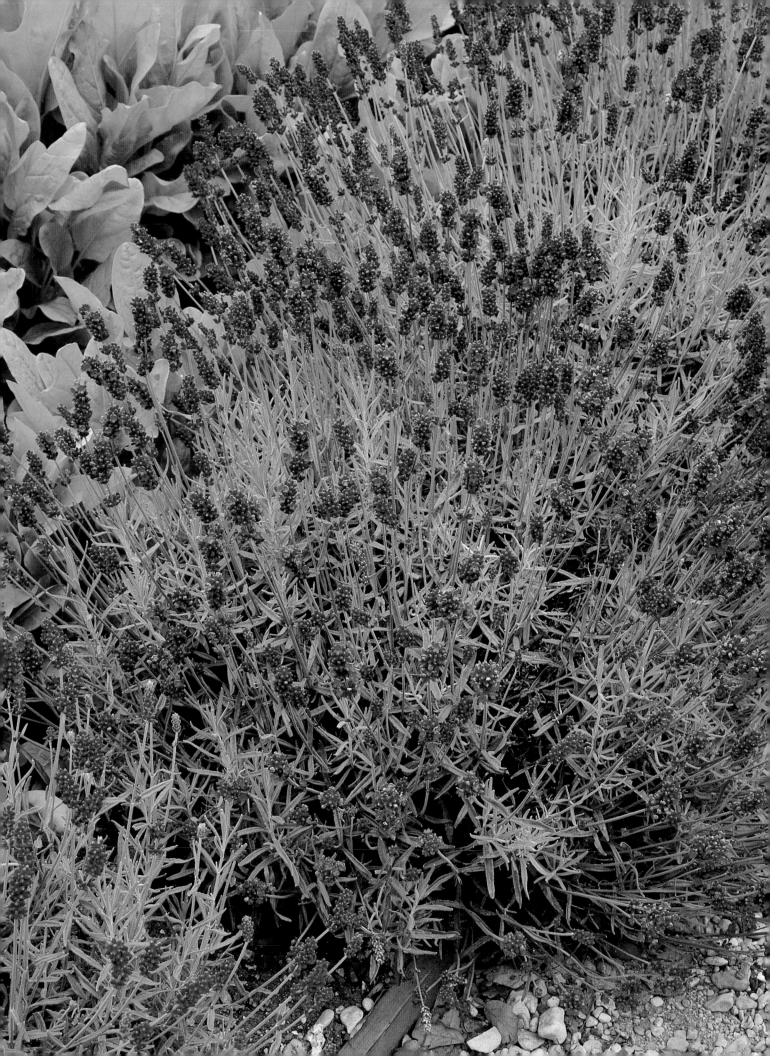

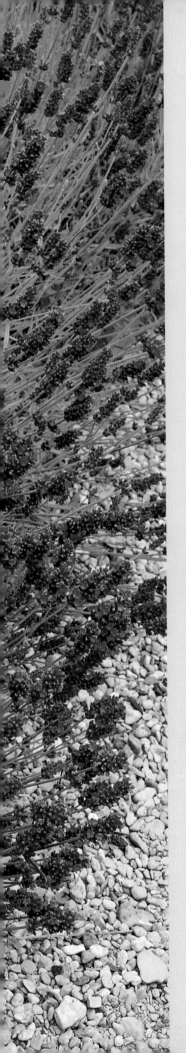

Contents

Introduction

There are no mysterious 'musts', no set rules, no finger of shame pointed at the gardener who doesn't follow an accepted pattern. Landscaping is not a complex and difficult art to be practised only by high priests.

THOMAS D CHURCH

Many of us are looking for ways to find relief from the everyday stresses of modern life. The mass of available self-help information, designed to enable us to improve our lot, sometimes feels as if it is having the opposite effect, as we struggle to achieve goals in our business, social and emotional lives. We crave time and space for relaxation and our homes can, and should, provide this sanctuary. Our gardens, no matter what their size, play a vital supporting role, affording release from the pressures of the outside world and helping to create a sense of personal fulfilment.

Real improvements to our environment often seem out of reach, yet a few simple techniques can help us in our ambition to lead healthier and happier lives. Several alternative approaches to health and well-being will be explored in this book, which aims to show how you can maximize the healing potential of your own garden.

Healthy bodies, healthy minds

Most people would agree that, despite all the scientific knowledge we have at our disposal, the general state of physical and mental well-being in Western society is pretty poor. There is obviously much more to health than being well fed and physically fit; the World Health Organization describes it as 'the condition of perfect bodily, spiritual and social well-being and not solely the absence of illness and injury'. Today, chronic illnesses and allergies are on the increase. Our constant battle against environmental pollution has led to our immune systems becoming worn down; this, in turn, has allowed serious diseases to gain a foothold. It is perhaps fortuitous that chronic illnesses, particularly those often considered incurable by conventional medicine, are the most likely to respond well to alternative methods.

There is currently an increased interest in holistic medicine throughout the West, with many people turning to complementary therapies such as

RIGHT Sitting in a garden brings you into contact with the healing power of nature. Even a public garden provides an opportunity to surround yourself with life-enhancing sunlight, the stabilizing influence of the earth and the all-embracing cycle of natural life.

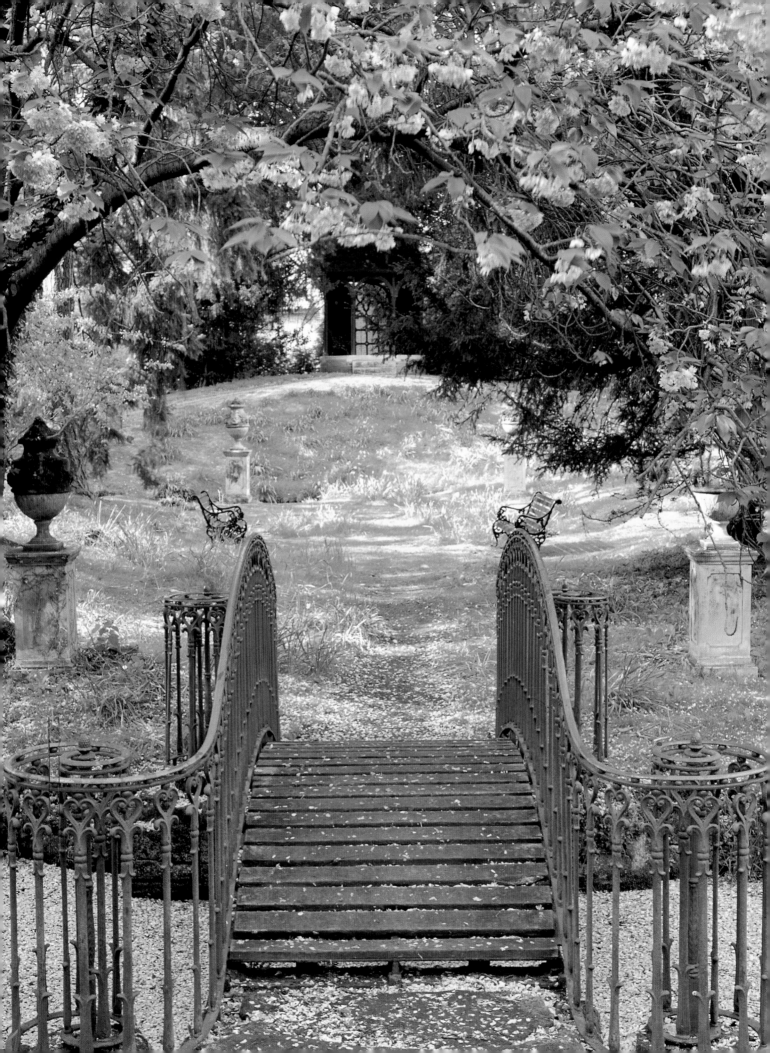

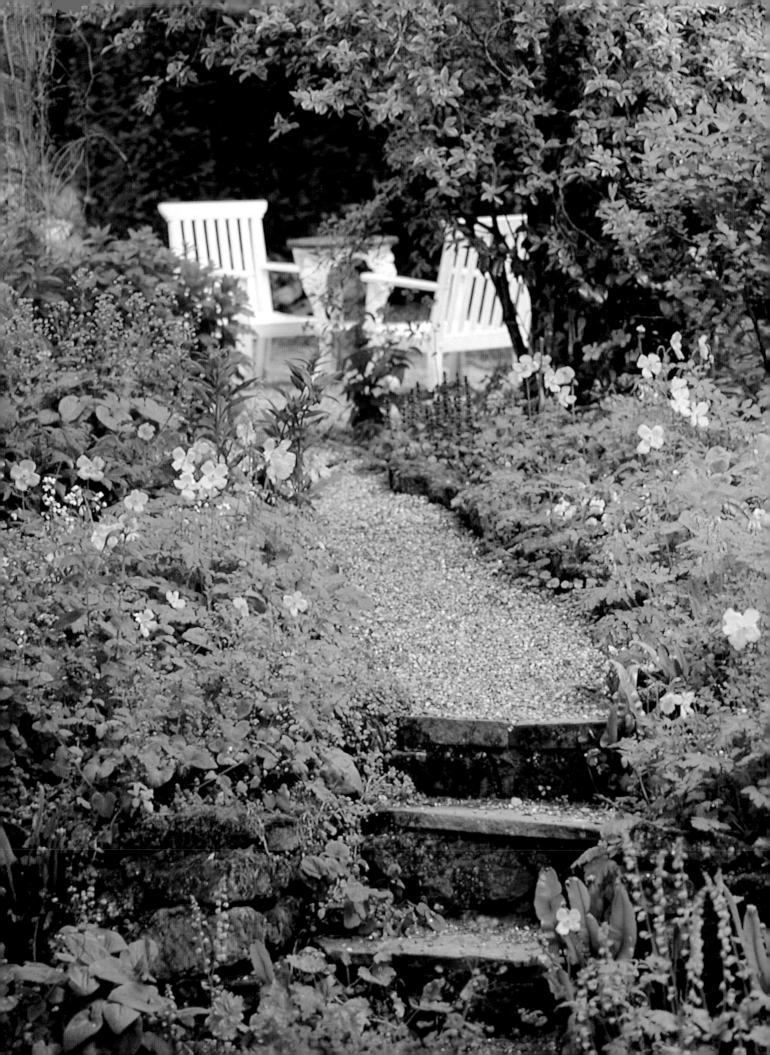

aromatherapy, feng shui, meditation and various approaches to herbalism. Whether this is due to ongoing research proving the efficacy of these practices, or to a general dissatisfaction with conventional medicine is hard to tell. However, at its best, alternative medicine should work in tandem with orthodox practice, imbuing it with a gentler, more intuitive approach.

From the beginning of time, many cultures have stressed the importance of balance within the individual for the maintenance of good health. All over the world, from North America to Australia, traditional societies continue to draw on the ancient wisdom of their ancestors for solutions to health and other problems. The practical use of natural materials is often combined with a deeply spiritual philosophy. The basis of holistic medicine is rooted in these cultures and continues to embrace the concept of 'the whole'.

Our bodies are complex entities and, according to holistic thinking, exist in a state where biochemistry is closely related to thoughts and emotions. Our hormones, reproductive cycle, sleep pattern, moods and metabolism are affected, to varying degrees, by our mental state. The most important systems are the endocrine, nervous and immune, which work together at many levels. Stress and emotional disharmony can upset the delicate balance of these systems and ultimately, therefore, the function of all body organs. This idea is relatively new to the West but, although still controversial in some quarters, acceptance is becoming more widespread. Our emotions have a profound effect upon our physical state and negative thought patterns are often reflected in the physical body. The good news is that if all disease has negativity behind it, ailments can be cured by reversing the mental patterns that fuel them. A happy mind creates a harmonious, and healthy, body – it is important to replace negative thoughts and emotions with positive, life-affirming ones.

A new science, psychoneuroimmunology, studies the link between stress and immune function, taking into account our individual methods of dealing with crisis. Certain discoveries have led to the conclusion that serious health problems can be caused by any prolonged disturbance of the mind/body equilibrium. This link between stress and ill health is of particular interest in such areas as cancer and AIDS research and, although treated with scepticism by many in conventional medicine, there is clear evidence that those who have suffered a loss or shock are more likely to be subsequently hospitalized through illness. The positive results of these studies are that certain psychological devices, such as relaxation and visualization exercises, can be of great benefit. Interestingly, research has also demonstrated that hospital patients recuperate more quickly when they have a view of an attractive outdoor environment.

Where conventional treatment aims for the speedy suppression of symptoms of illness (and acceptance of unpleasant side effects), natural healing requires a little more patience as it takes time for the body to heal itself. Holistic practitioners look to the causes and prevention of illness rather than simply the control of symptoms.

Lasting cures demand that the patient accepts responsibility for the healing process. By looking more closely at your lifestyle, you may well discover patterns that prevent you from functioning at your best and contribute to any health problems that you may have. Your thoughts and feelings are as likely to be at the root of your problem as diet and environment. Due to the individual nature of such influences, in holistic terms, people with the same apparent illness may have very different causes and therefore need to follow a different treatment path.

Perseverance and observation are required in order to allow our bodies time to adjust to more subtle treatments, and to assess the changes that they bring about. By cultivating a stronger immune system and stimulating the body's natural defences through a better balanced lifestyle, you will become more responsive to the relatively gentle healing vibrations around you. There are countless opportunities for self-help and it doesn't matter which technique you adopt, as long as it suits you. Find out a little more about meditation, colour healing, aromatherapy or feng shui ... and take the plunge!

LEFT In your own garden you can indulge all your senses: choose plants that appeal to you for their colour or shape, their smell or texture; sip your morning coffee or a cool drink while you listen to the sounds of birdsong and rustling leaves.

Sanctuary in the garden

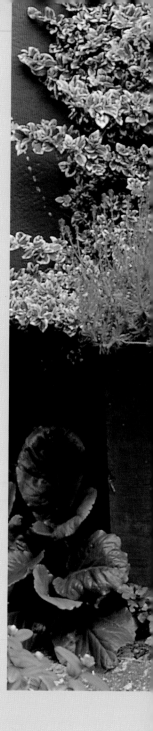

The primary aim of this book is to demonstrate how to turn the garden into a therapeutic environment where we can reduce the pace of life in order to de-stress our life. The sensory overload of work, traffic, child-rearing and shopping can be replaced by a gentler stimulation of the senses, concentrating on those aspects which are so often ignored in our race to get through each day.

We need to spend time 'being', and not just 'doing', and the garden offers an ideal opportunity for relaxation. This does mean, however, that it cannot be viewed as just another generator of mundane chores. Instead, we should learn to think of it as a haven where we can be embraced by the natural world.

In the quest for total health, we must nurture all aspects of our life, including the spiritual. Often neglected, it is perhaps the most important of all in terms of good health and when ignored, our life can seem superficial and meaningless. Simple meditation will bring us more in touch with our inner selves. Guidance on using the garden as a focal point is given in Chapter 6, Meditation.

Above all else, the garden is a perfect place for self expression, a place where you can be creative, developing aspects of your self which may be denied elsewhere in your life. If it makes you happy, introduce an element of humour into the garden, a feature that makes you smile every time you see it. There is more than a grain of truth in the old saying 'laughter is the best medicine', and pleasure has an important role to play in healing.

The power of nature

There is something about the constant cycle of growth and change that is utterly absorbing. Gardening helps you to get back to basics and provides an escape from everyday problems.

We have much to gain from regular contact with the natural world, whether in terms of feeling more 'grounded', or through the plants we choose to grow and the wildlife that they will attract. Anyone who spends time in their garden will be aware of the healing powers of nature and the freeing sensation of feeling a connection with the earth. Many of us today live in surroundings that are almost totally isolated from any natural habitat, yet we were never designed to live in such sterile conditions.

In recent decades, 24-hour lighting and heating has detached us from the cyclical rhythms of day, month and year that mark the passage of time. An awareness of the transience of the seasons is beneficial to all of us and may be particularly helpful for sufferers of Seasonal Affective Disorder. This problem, causing lethargy and sometimes severe depression during the winter months, has been linked to a lack of natural light. In order to feel more closely attuned to nature's cycles, aim to spend more time outside. Get into the garden at every opportunity, day and night, and really look for the changes: differences in light level and tone, the height of the sun, the changing shape of the moon. This time dimension separates garden design from every other art form; our gardens are never completely finished, having both good and bad moments because of the all-embracing influence of nature.

When you plan for seasonal effect, visualize the garden throughout the year and aim to exploit the full glory of each season. Although we may not be fully aware of it, we associate distinct colours and activities with certain times of the year. Spring brings an explosion of colour, through the greens of young foliage and a myriad of bulbs and early shrubs in light and cheerful colours, mostly yellows and blues. A time of great activity, we sow seeds, plant up containers, cut the grass and have a general clear-out.

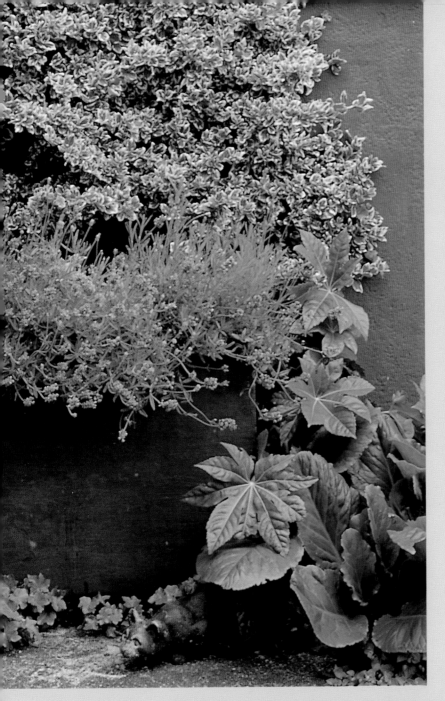

And so it begins again, drawing us along in its wake, promising a rebirth with every death and always better things to come.

Gardeners know that to have a beautiful garden they must have a caring touch. Although we may seem to be rigorously controlling and manipulating nature, every garden will fail without a hefty dose of tender loving care.

In order to make life easier for yourself, aim to work with nature, rather than against it, whenever you can. Embrace the materials you have at your disposal to create not a contrived garden, but an improved version of nature, in order to invoke the spirit of the place. It makes no sense to attempt to grow azaleas on an alkaline soil or Mediterranean plants on heavy clay; any alterations you make will only temporarily modify existing conditions. You will save time, effort, money and disappointment by first studying where a plant comes from and then providing conditions as similar as possible to those of its native habitat. If something you want to grow is simply not cut out for your soil conditions or climate, make another choice; there are, after all, thousands of possibilities.

Our gardens are a microcosm of the universe and we need to take a more holistic view – on both a personal and global scale. Many aspects of our environment are extremely unhealthy and our everyday actions cause yet more damage to the earth. It surely goes without saying that any steps we take to improve conditions for the inhabitants of our gardens will also inevitably create a healthier environment for us.

We need to acquire respect for the earth and adopt a 'sustainable' approach towards everything we do, so that future generations are protected from our potentially damaging actions. Plants play a vital role in healing the planet, supporting the atmosphere through their natural processes and contributing to a more healthy environment. Through an 'environmentally friendly' attitude and an awareness of 'sustainability', no matter how humble our garden, we should feel connected to the earth in the broadest possible sense.

ABOVE The foliage of *Bergenia cordifolia* and *Fatsia japonica* in this corner partially conceals a stalking stone cat – your garden should bring you pleasure, so include items that make you smile.

In summer there is another burst of colour, this time more potent, the warmth of the sun bringing out every shade imaginable and building up to the rich hues of the late summer border. We are kept busy mowing, weeding and deadheading yet still find the time to enjoy the weather (fingers crossed!).

Acting as a grand finale to the gardening year, autumn goes out with a bang, full of fiery shades – rich reds, oranges and russets. Once we have gathered in the harvest and tidied everything up, we put the garden to bed for a while, relying only on a few winter-flowering bulbs and shrubs for their transient display. The muted winter palette of pale grass, weak sunlight and bare soil takes hold and life lies dormant, albeit waiting just beneath the surface.

Gardening for the senses

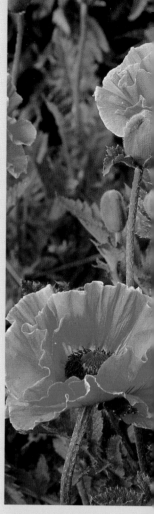

Gardens should be stimulating environments – both mentally and physically – and can be designed to provide a rich sensory experience. Sight tends to dominate, but sometimes all you need to do is close your eyes and wait for the other senses to wake up and provide an unexpected new appreciation of the garden you never knew you had! Touch, sight, sound, smell and taste can all be catered for and each has a significant role to play in maintaining health. Sight is dealt with primarily in the chapter on Colour therapy; smell in Aromatherapy; taste in the chapters on Herbalism and Holistic Gardening. The remaining two senses, touch and sound, are equally important and have a special role to play in gardens for the blind and partially sighted.

Touch

In almost any garden there is a wealth of sensations simply waiting to be discovered, and a great deal to be said for taking your gardening gloves off once in a while and getting to grips with the garden *au naturel*! As long as you are not handling dangerous or irritant materials (see page 32), you should come to little harm. Intimate contact with your surroundings will help to finely tune your tactile senses. For those who tend to shy away from such contact, simply make an effort to touch the plants and other surfaces in your garden; you will be amazed at the variety of sensations you encounter. Use not only your hands but also other parts of your body, such as your feet or face. In texture alone, plants offer an enormous variety of sensory experience, yet this is, to date, a much under-exploited facet of gardening.

Some trees have wonderful bark textures which draw you closer, inviting your touch. The trunks of a cork oak (*Quercus suber*), mature pear (*Pyrus communis)* and sweet chestnut (*Castanea sativa*) are deeply fissured and demand further investigation with probing fingers. Snakebark maples (*Acer capillipes, A. grosseri* and *A. rufinerve*) have a fascinating covering which is strangely self-patterned yet smooth to the touch. Many trees shed their bark (*Acer griseum, Eucalyptus* spp., *Betula papyrifera, Platanus x hispanica*) and you can't help but give nature a hand by peeling off a few sheets. A few simply defy belief, such as the bark of *Sequoiadendron giganteum*, which is so soft and spongy you can push your fingers right into it. Finally, there are those which are unusually smooth and glossy such as *Prunus serrula*; plant them near a path where you can stroke them as you pass by.

Most people are aware of the furry 'lambs' ears' of *Stachys byzantina* or male catkins of pussy willow (*Salix* spp.). The same texture can be experienced in the leaves of *Verbascum olympicum, Hydrangea aspera* subsp. *sargentiana, Ballota pseudodictamnus, Buddleja crispa, Lavandula lanata, Salvia argentea* and *Pelargonium tomentosum*.

Foliage can be smooth and bold, inviting a passing touch (canna, *Hosta* cvs., *Magnolia grandiflora*), or prickly, dissuading you from getting too close (*Gunnera manicata, Ilex aquifolium, Rubus* spp.). Feathery leaves are worth growing for their delicate texture (fennel, many ferns, artemisia, most cut-leafed species), as are ornamental grasses (*Pennisetum orientale, Festuca glauca, Stipa gigantea*). Some foliage is sticky from resins or strangely waxy (*Cistus* spp., *Lavandula* spp., *Crambe cordifolia*) and a few leaves even have a unique quilted finish as they unfurl (*Rodgersia* spp., *Veratrum* spp.).

Flowers also have an important part to play in the sensuous garden, from the tiniest, daintiest heads of *Alchemilla mollis* through to monsters such as sunflowers. Individual petals often have a luxurious,

ABOVE The hairy buds of the oriental poppy, *Papaver orientale* 'Suleika', open to reveal silky, strokable petals.

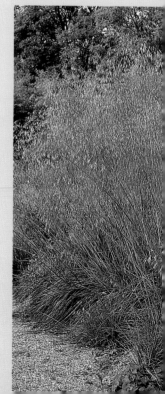

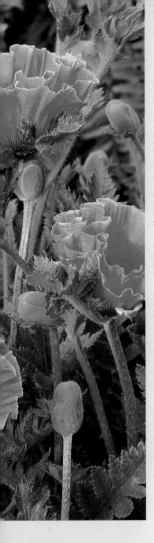

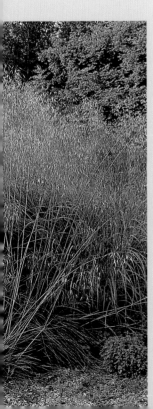

BELOW Listen to the whispering of *Stipa gigantea* (feather grass) and the contrasting crunch of gravel.

satiny sheen, like the oriental poppies or large daisies such as *Helenium* or *Cosmos* spp. The dangling flower heads of bleeding heart (*Dicentra spectabilis*) or angel's fishing rod (*Dierama pulcherrimum*) seem perfectly balanced when cupped in the hand while the globes of *Allium* or *Echinops* spp. draw attention with their incredible symmetry, as does the almost unnatural flatness of *Achillea filipendulina* and some of the *Sedum* spp.

There are even flowers that invite play; who doesn't remember making snapdragons 'snap'? I know that neither of these should be encouraged, but I vividly remember wearing individual foxglove flowers on my fingers as a child and delighting at the 'pop' of a fuchsia bud when I squashed it!

When the flowers are over, many seeds continue to provide sensory stimulation. Often considered a menace in gardens, the seedpods of Himalayan balsam (*Impatiens glandulifera*) explode when touched, torpedoing the seeds far and wide. Ever popular with children and flower arrangers are honesty, with its papery, translucent seedheads, and poppy capsules, with their delicate, brittle quality. Some seeds even cover themselves in silky hairs and are remarkably soft to the touch; these include *Pulsatilla vulgaris* and many varieties of clematis.

Sound

Wherever possible, gardens should provide a refuge from the noise pollution and disturbances of everyday life. Living with the daily stress of unwelcome noise, we often forget about the value of sound in our gardens, only becoming aware of 'noise' when it is intrusive, such as next door's radio or lawnmower. However, we can design the more pleasing aspects of sound into the garden to introduce an extra dimension and generate a positive mood. Even items such as wind chimes can bring pleasure and instil a feeling of tranquillity.

The sound of rain – as long as you are not caught out in it – can be very refreshing. This is an ancient concept: for many centuries, Chinese scholars planted large-leafed plants beneath their windows, in order to emphasize the pattering sound.

Rainfall may be uncontrollable but its sound can be mimicked by installing moving water in the garden. Water features can be designed to fit any space and create all manner of sounds, from the gentle tinkling of a fountain or the gushing of a powerful waterfall to the rhythmic motion of a Japanese bird scarer and the bubbling of a small geyser. Such features are best sited out of the prevailing wind and their output may need to be adjusted in order to achieve the desired sound. Even a still pool has the capacity to make noises as fish rise to the surface or a frog plops into the water.

The movement of wind through trees and shrubs also produces refreshing sounds and some species are particularly effective in a breeze, especially the softly rustling bamboos and grasses. The following are useful for providing gentle background noise:

Briza media (QUAKING GRASS)
Colutea arborescens (BLADDER SENNA)
Cortaderia selloana (PAMPAS GRASS)
Eucalyptus spp. (GUM TREE)
Fargesia nitida (BAMBOO)
Fraxinus ornus (MANNA ASH)
Lunaria annua (HONESTY)
Miscanthus spp.
Molinia caerulea (MOOR GRASS)
Papaver spp. (POPPY SEEDHEADS)
Phormium tenax (NEW ZEALAND FLAX)
Phyllostachys nigra (BLACK BAMBOO)
Picea breweriana (BREWER'S WEEPING SPRUCE)
Populus tremula (ASPEN)
Salix spp. (WILLOWS)
Stipa gigantea (FEATHER GRASS)

The hum of bees and other insects on a warm day can be almost hypnotic, although you sometimes need to be quite still to tune into this most gentle of sounds. Birdsong is also a delight, and through your efforts to attract insect life and to make your garden 'green', you should find more birds will be attracted than ever before. For details of tactics to attract bees, birds and other wildlife into your garden, turn to Chapter 1, Holistic gardening.

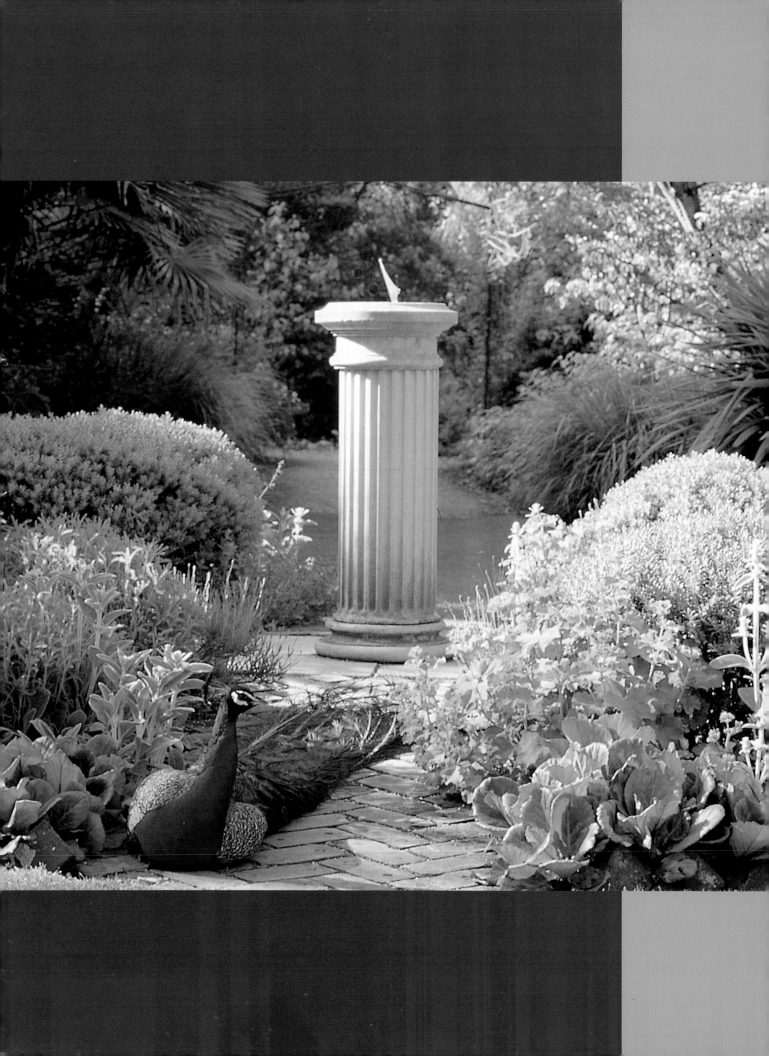

1

Holistic gardening

Each particle is a matter of immensity;
each leaf a world;
each insect an inexplicable compendium.

JOHANN KASPAR LAVATER

The holistic philosophy, that the whole is greater than the sum of its parts, can be applied to gardening at many levels. At its most basic, it is clear that healthy earth and water are needed to produce healthy plants, which in turn support a wide range of wildlife. Multiplied many times, the principles of nature's food chains have far-reaching consequences. In concentrating on our own little patch of earth, we can create a microcosm with diverse habitats that can make a positive contribution to the health of the entire planet. Whether or not you aim to attract birds and butterflies, their presence is a sign of life and growth in your garden. Seen another way, this means that instead of simply treating the individual problems we encounter in our gardens (whether aphids, black spot or poor plant growth) we need to consider the whole garden. This is the fundamental logic behind organic gardening.

We take our own place in the food chain when we grow fruit, vegetables and herbs, and later in this chapter we shall look at the ways in which even the smallest garden can produce delicious and useful crops.

In order to enjoy good health we need to live in a beneficial environment, yet these days our immediate surroundings are often threatened by a host of potential dangers. In addition to the problems we individually and collectively bring upon ourselves through air pollution and the use of dangerous chemicals and materials, there are also hazards initiated by nature itself. Some problems can be controlled through a more open-minded approach to the gardens we create. Air pollution, for example, can be tackled first of all by growing certain plants that can positively improve air quality, and ensuring that they remain healthy. Air quality is also affected by dust, fungal spores and pollen: these natural pollutants bring misery to allergy sufferers, but, again, their effects can be greatly reduced by appropriate garden management, careful plant selection and the creation of a low-allergen garden. Many health risks can be mitigated by so-called 'green' practices; risk limitation starts with the adoption of an organic regime.

LEFT Few gardens can entertain peacocks, but by adopting an organic approach you will encourage other feathered visitors which will bring as much pleasure.

15

Organic gardening

Organic gardening requires a holistic approach and a frame of mind that views the garden as a whole. Managing the garden organically will inevitably lead to the development of a more balanced environment which will be supportive of its inhabitants. It helps to bear in mind that every action produces a reaction.

The first consideration for the organic gardener is the exclusion of any products that are not derived from natural sources – which includes many popular garden products. Some of these are used directly to treat plants, such as inorganic fertilizers, pesticides and herbicides, but there is also a vast range of peripheral garden chemicals which remain in many people's horticultural arsenal. For example, creosote is believed to be potentially carcinogenic, yet is regularly used to protect outdoor timber, and tanalized (pressure treated) timber is treated with heavy metals and poisons (copper, chrome and arsenic) which may have the potential to cause as yet unforeseen problems.

Soil

Your garden is shaped by environmental conditions such as soil, aspect and climate; each needs to be taken into account to ensure you are adopting a suitable approach. Many would argue that the most vital element in an organic garden is the soil and that it needs to be considered as a living organism in its own right. You will be more than repaid for any attention you lavish upon it. Good soil structure supports strong plant growth, which leads to natural resistance, and this in itself is probably more important than any other cultural improvements you might make.

The incorporation of bulky organic matter is most beneficial and it is almost impossible to overdo. Good garden compost or well-rotted animal manures are suitable, as are a wide range of other materials, from composted seaweed to leaf mould and spent mushroom compost. Organic gardeners even bury banana skins, old leather shoes and horsehair mattresses to provide nutrients as they rot down! All these materials will help to improve soil structure through aeration. Light, sandy soils will benefit from the incorporation of nutrient-rich humus and will achieve better water retention, while heavier clay soils will become more free-draining and therefore easier to work.

Every gardener, whether organic or not, should try to find space for a compost bin. Through recycling suitable garden and household waste, not only can you reduce the burden on local waste disposal systems but you will also be provided with a valuable, and free, soil additive. Composting is not a complicated recipe – make it part of your everyday life, adding eggshells, teabags, vegetable peelings (not meat scraps, because they are likely to attract rats), dead pot plants and their potting medium, as well as grass clippings and other garden waste.

For an effective yet tidy compost bin, begin with a wire cage or basket or other open structure to allow some air to circulate round it. To speed up the process and ensure adequate aeration, turn the heap with a garden fork once or twice during composting. The area can be disguised with an outer frame or screened by a leafy plant.

If space is really at a premium, or you want to see more rapid results, you might consider a worm bin. Although you can buy these in 'kit' form, even down to the mail-order worms, a dustbin with holes drilled in the bottom will also do the trick. Simply keep the contents damp and frost-free and top up regularly with everyday kitchen waste. You will be rewarded with a nutrient-rich compost and often also a liquid feed which can be drawn off separately.

Manures and composts will build up the soil's

nutrient status so that there will be less need to resort to chemical fertilizers. When applied to moist soil as a deep mulch, compost will also suppress weed growth and retain moisture throughout the growing season, both of which reduce the stresses on plants, leading to healthier growth. By reducing the amount of irrigation required and thus saving water, you will also be protecting the wider environment. Further steps in this direction include installing a water butt and re-using washing-up water.

To prevent permanent damage to the soil structure, care should be taken over the timing of certain garden operations. Heavy soils in particular should never be walked on when wet. Some organic gardeners even practise 'no dig' techniques and keep off the ground completely, relying solely on deep mulches of organic matter to improve soil structure through the action of earthworms.

Weed control

Many people find that one downside to an organic approach is the issue of weeds. Although hoeing and hand weeding are effective at keeping them at bay, always aim to disturb the soil as little as possible, otherwise you will bring more seeds to the surface where they can more readily germinate. Make life easier for yourself by working with the weather – hoeing in dry, sunny weather will kill weeds off before they can re-root on the surface.

An important technique is never to allow ground to lay idle or unplanted. Dense ground-cover planting and mulches are the best methods of keeping weeds in check. If land is being 'rested' for some reason, either between crops or in preparation for new shrub plantings, ensure it is entirely covered. This might be with a mulch of chipped bark, black polythene or old carpet. For longer periods, a 'green' manure crop such as fenugreek, alfalfa or annual lupins can be grown and then dug in at the end of its life cycle, returning important nutrients to the soil. Rotted nettles also make an excellent green manure.

It is inevitable, however, that these methods will involve more effort than a single herbicide application. Where every minute of a hectic life is

precious, there are those who feel life is too short to justify the hours spent tackling bindweed armed with nothing more than a garden fork. If you simply cannot live without weedkiller, at least ensure you follow the manufacturer's instructions to the letter and choose one that is as 'environmentally friendly' as possible. The same rules apply when a serious infestation of pests occurs – choose a problem-specific product which will do the least possible harm to the 'good' garden bugs.

It may go against all you have ever held dear but weeds do have their uses. Many provide important food sources for native fauna and some, dare I say it, are even attractive in their own right. Consider the highly desirable 'wildflower meadow'; what is it if not a collection of weeds grown through grass? Learn, if you can, to tolerate at least a few uninvited visitors and if you feel you are losing control and it is all about to get the better of you, don't panic. Concentrate your immediate efforts on those weeds that are on the verge of flowering, since the old chestnut 'one year's seed is seven years' weed' is, unfortunately, well founded!

Garden materials

Some organic issues have an effect far beyond your own garden; when choosing materials, try to select those of natural origin. Clay pavers, stone flags, timber and terracotta are all preferable to concrete or plastic alternatives, the production of which can devastate natural resources and increase pollution. There is just one proviso: if using stone in any form, buy from a reclaimed source wherever possible. Avoid weathered rockery stone at all costs unless you can be absolutely certain that it hasn't been taken directly from a natural source. Our few remaining native river ecologies and limestone pavements need all the protection they can get.

For the same reason, take care when buying timber furniture and ensure the wood has been taken from a managed plantation. Finally, it almost goes without saying that we should opt for non-peat based composts such as coir in order to conserve the world's threatened peat bogs.

Garden pests

Pests and diseases can present the organic gardener with many problems. Most, however, can be prevented through good hygiene, cultural controls and the selection of disease-immune varieties. Some shrubs and trees are naturally more resistant to attacks from pests and diseases, and other plants, such as roses and many vegetable varieties, have had disease resistance bred into them. If all else fails, there are some acceptable organic sprays available commercially, but even these should be used sparingly. Interestingly, an infusion of horsetail (*Equisetum*) and stinging nettle is said to remove aphids and other pests from most plants.

Gardening organically will, over time, encourage a natural balance to establish in the garden; an increase in pests should be followed by a rise in the numbers of natural predators. This does mean, however, that you have to accept a permanent low level pest presence so that there is a corresponding food source for predators at all times.

Thriving colonies of ladybirds, hoverflies and lacewings (which eat aphids, mites and other pests), ground beetles and centipedes (which eat slugs and vine weevils), frogs, thrushes and hedgehogs will all wage war against unwanted visitors. Not only should you avoid broad-spectrum pesticides, but you will also need to provide habitats, in terms of both food sources and shelter, for their ongoing survival. Do not tidy the garden so much in late autumn that it is left completely bare, as dead plants and crevices in log piles are used by many animals to overwinter.

For plants that require specific protection from attack, there are useful physical barriers which keep pests away. These include greasebands and pheromone traps for fruit trees to prevent damage by various moths; paper collars on brassicas to prevent the cabbage root fly burrowing into the soil to lay eggs; fine horticultural fleece over carrots to keep out the carrot root fly. Some pests can be effectively controlled through very simple means – slugs and caterpillars are easily picked off by hand. If this is beyond you, beer traps are an efficient option: a saucer or jam jar full of beer will lure them to their death – by drowning while intoxicated! Sawdust, grit, ash and oak leaves placed around susceptible plants will also discourage slugs and snails.

Before arming yourself with any chemical, first consider your available options; there are many controls that have no long-term health implications. For instance, earwig infestations can devastate some flowering plants but are readily controlled by simple traps, so why use chemicals? Woodlice may be annoying but they don't generally damage anything, so is it really necessary to kill them?

Apply this rule to every garden problem; a little thought and investigation will often serve up a less damaging alternative. The decision to go organic will inevitably mean occasional holes in leaves and even the loss of a plant now and then. Such 'failures' can be hard to accept in a world where we constantly strive for perfection. But over the longer term, the benefits must outweigh the losses and if we can play even a small part in making our world a healthier place in which to live, it has to be worthwhile.

Companion planting

Some pests can be successfully controlled through companion planting – the use of certain plants which, when planted near others, have a deterrent effect upon their known pests. Some companion plants are believed to excrete chemicals which the pests or diseases dislike. Examples include chives (and other members of the *Allium* or onion family, such as the increasingly popular ornamentals) controlling black spot on roses; nasturtium controlling woolly aphid and whitefly; French marigolds preventing blackfly attack; onions and rosemary deterring carrot root fly. Hyssop attracts cabbage butterflies away from cabbage crops, and many strongly scented herbs such as sage and mint will deter a whole variety of pests and so are especially valuable.

Growing plants in mixed groups as opposed to massed schemes of one genus is also effective and applies equally to ornamental plantings and fruit or vegetables. The different plants provide mutual protection from pests since a serious infestation is less likely to build up in the first place.

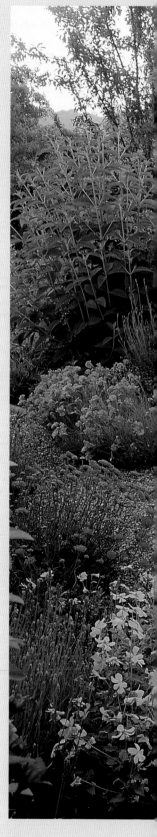

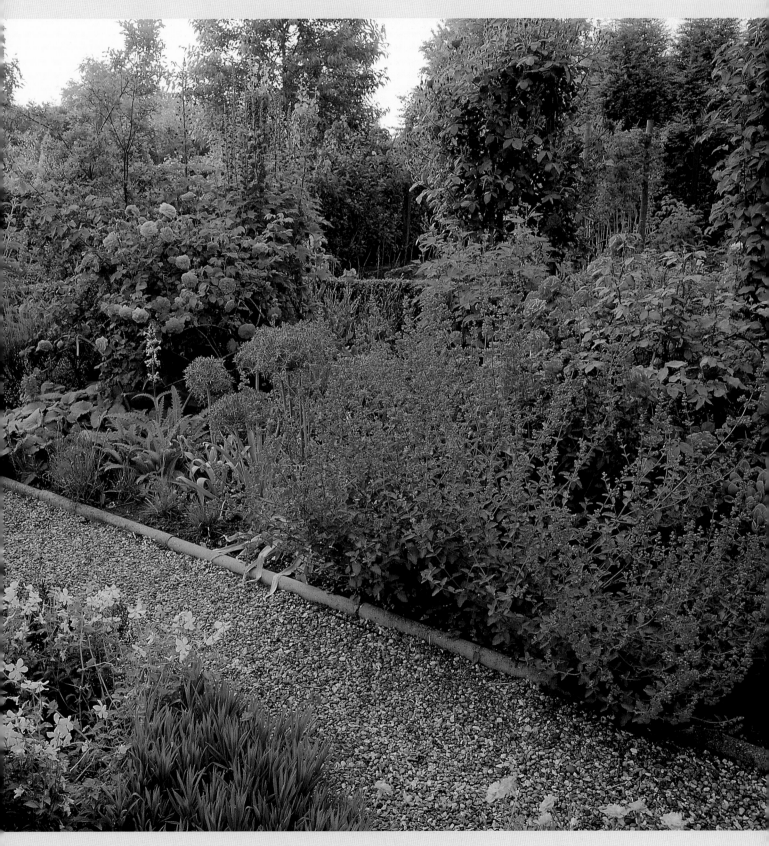

Wildlife gardening

There are at least two good reasons to encourage wildlife into your garden. First, many insects, birds and mammals are very efficient pest controllers and, if you adopt an organic approach, will assist in the war against unwanted guests. Secondly, an important aspect of gardening is the enjoyment of fauna as well as flora in your garden. Who hasn't delighted at the sight of a *Buddleja* smothered in butterflies, a blue tit dangling from the catkins of a birch, or an unexpected clump of frogspawn in a tiny urban pond? If your garden is filled with bees, butterflies, birds and other visiting animals, you can be sure that the environment is beneficial and supportive of you as well as them.

This sort of contact with nature can provide a vital release from our sterile, stressful lives and bring us back in touch with our wider surroundings. Almost any plant in a garden will attract a bee or some other insect, even if it simply investigates, then disappears again. Putting out bird food in winter encourages birds into even a concrete-clad garden. You will often find that such simple steps bring in a surprisingly high number of visitors. If, however, you live in what you feel is an utterly barren environment and hardly ever see a living creature (other than next door's cat), you still have options. Try to escape to a bit of open space every so often to 'feed' that part of your life which is missing and you will, no doubt, feel uplifted. This doesn't need to be the depths of some unspoilt countryside; even a walk in your local park will have the desired effect.

To encourage the widest range of wild creatures into your garden, you need to view it as a miniature nature reserve. Where space allows, your aim should be to establish a species-rich environment with as many diverse areas of natural habitat as possible. Try to adapt to your local ecology and use the ideas on the following pages to establish a range of habitats, according to the space available in your own garden. However, even the smallest border can include plants that have been chosen especially to attract butterflies.

Bear in mind that the decision to make the garden a sanctuary from harmful pesticides is infinitely more important than the number of plants you include. Traces of chemicals have the potential to poison the many tiny inhabitants of our gardens that provide a feast for creatures higher up the food chain, such as birds and hedgehogs. Other things you can do in a garden of any size is to leave stumps or logs as habitats for predatory insects such as centipedes and ground beetles, and put up nesting boxes for birds.

Whatever you aim to attract into your garden, you need to embrace an alternative concept of tidiness. To have a supportive, species-rich environment, you have to loosen your grip a little:

- Don't remove every dead flower towards the end of the summer – seedheads are a very important food source in winter.
- Don't mow every area of grass to within an inch of its life – longer grass shelters and supports a myriad of wildlife.
- Include a log pile to provide an overwintering site.
- Try to leave a few weeds in an unnoticeable spot – they are immensely valuable to all forms of wildlife (remove the flower heads before they go to seed, to prevent them taking over the entire garden).
- Don't feel you have to cultivate every bit of ground – letting nature take over a small part of your garden is likely to repay you with a fascinating inflow of wildlife.
- Remember to take care when tidying up in early spring to avoid unnecessarily disturbing over-wintering animals in any of the above areas.

RIGHT *Buddleja* is well known for its ability to attract butterflies, so much so that its common name is butterfly bush.

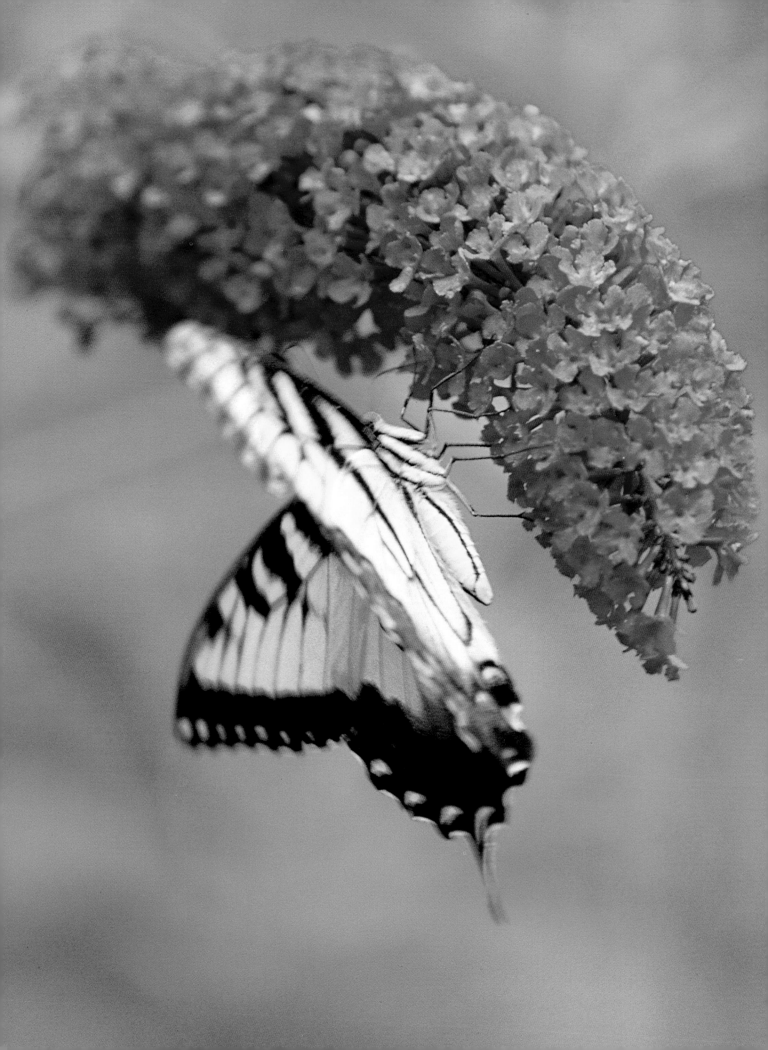

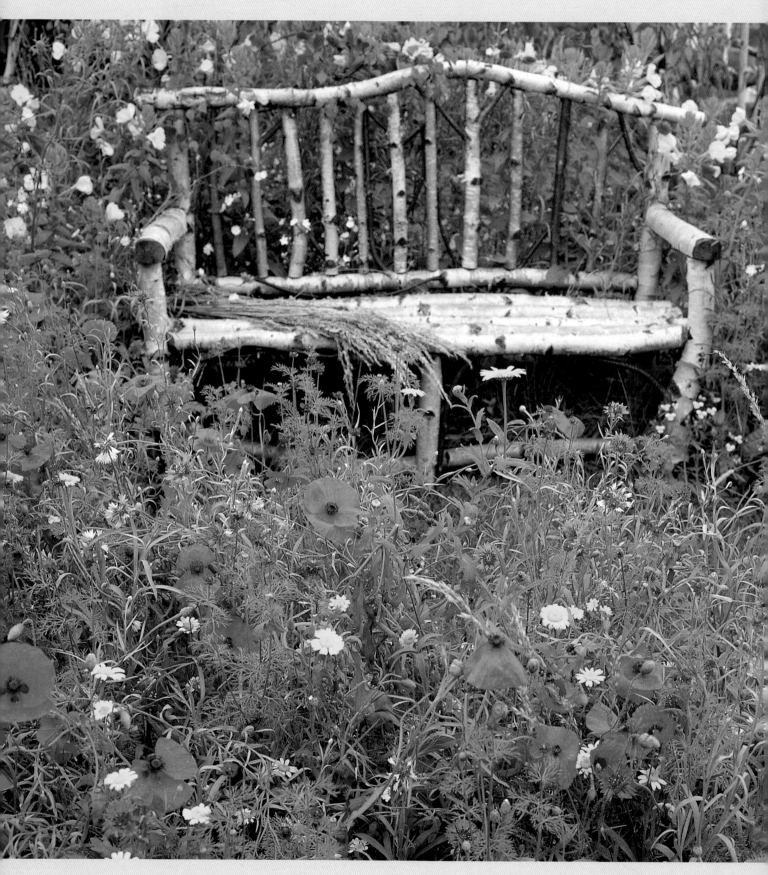

LEFT Poppies and cornflowers self-seed readily, while other plants, such as oxeye daisies, will grow as perennials to appear year after year in your wildflower meadow.

Wildflower meadow

Almost any area of grass can be enhanced by the inclusion of a few wildflowers, which will lighten up a potentially dull area with a kaleidoscope of colour. There is also value in leaving some grass longer, as it provides winter cover for insects and small animals and is a useful food source in autumn.

Although it is impossible to truly replicate an ancient hay meadow in your garden, it is surprisingly easy to create a fair imitation. Your soil type and aspect needs to be investigated, be it acid or alkaline, wet or dry, sunny or shady, so that suitable plants can be selected from what may initially seem an overwhelming list. To establish a wildflower meadow from scratch, a proprietary seed mix can be sown directly on to soil (preferably with a low nutrient status) and initially cultivated much as any 'normal' grassed area. Regular mowing in the first year allows the plants to establish while keeping the grass in check; early flowers are sacrificed for stronger vegetative growth. Alternatively, for an established lawn, or to make life a little easier, plant small 'plugs' of native plants directly into the sward.

Where this type of grassland differs from an ordinary lawn is over the issue of maintenance. Although a wildflower meadow is less demanding and need only be mown a few times each year, it is advisable to do so more often, if only to prevent the grass swamping the flowers. Do not assume such areas can be left entirely to their own devices; rank 'weeds' such as docks and nettles greatly appreciate neglect and will predominate if not controlled.

The best result is likely to be obtained with summer-flowering species as this offers the widest choice of suitable plants and simplifies the management regime. However, this means that spring-flowering plants such as cowslip will be excluded, as they will suffer from being treated in the same manner as later-flowering plants. Summer meadows should be left to grow unhindered through the spring and during flowering and seed-setting before being cut in August. They can then be mown regularly until the end of the season to keep them tidy.

If space is really at a premium in your garden, many of these plants can be grown in a small annual border, creating the illusion of a meadow without the maintenance requirements of grass.

The following temperate plants grow on most soils and are tolerant of varied conditions; for specific areas such as woodland, boggy, or dry calcareous soil, seek advice from a reputable seed house. Where possible, try to use seed of local provenance, so that the genetic profile of native plants in your area is not affected by cross pollination.

Meadow plants

Achillea millefolium (YARROW)
Agrimonia eupatoria (AGRIMONY)
Campanula rotundifolia (HAREBELL)
Centauria cyanus (CORNFLOWER)
Galium verum (LADY'S BEDSTRAW)
Geranium pratense (MEADOW CRANESBILL)
Knautia arvensis (FIELD SCABIOUS)
Leucanthemum vulgare (OXEYE DAISY)
Linaria vulgaris (COMMON TOADFLAX)
Linum perenne (PERENNIAL FLAX)
Lotus corniculatus (BIRD'S-FOOT TREFOIL)
Lychnis flos-cuculi (RAGGED ROBIN)
Malva moschata (MUSK MALLOW)
Papaver rhoeas (CORN POPPY)
Primula vulgaris (PRIMROSE)
Prunella vulgaris (SELFHEAL)
Rhinanthus minor (YELLOW RATTLE)
Silene dioica (RED CAMPION)
Stachys officinalis (BETONY)
Vicia sativa (COMMON VETCH)

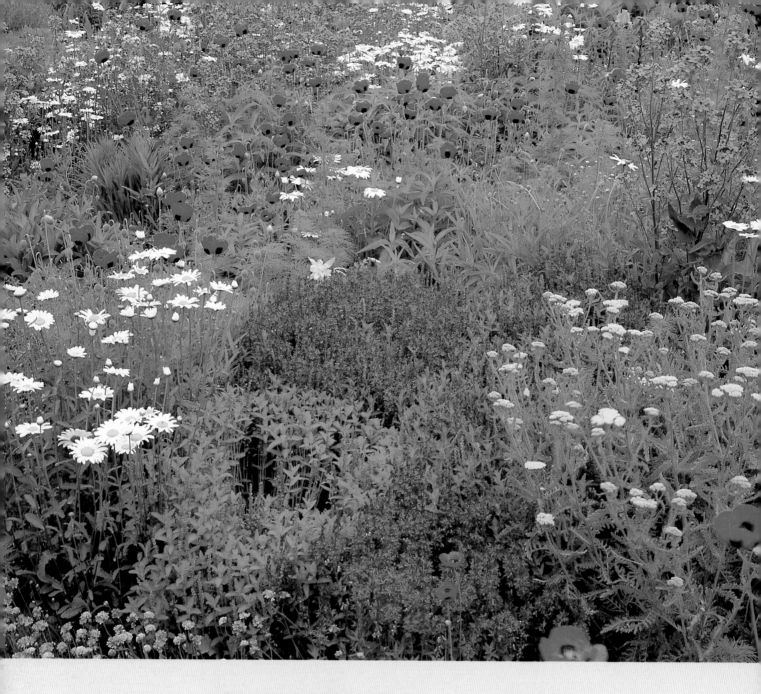

Attracting butterflies, bees and other insects

Invite these little creatures into your garden by offering them a source of food – plants rich in pollen or nectar – ideally in a sunny, sheltered spot where they can settle easily on the flowers without being buffeted by the wind. Although most flowers will attract insects, open flowers (particularly in yellow and white) such as *Leucanthemum vulgare* (oxeye daisy), *Limnanthes douglasii* (poached egg plant), *Nemophila menziesii* (baby blue-eyes) and *Chamaemelum nobile* (chamomile) are favoured by hoverflies, as are *Achillea millefolium* (yarrow), *Scabiosa* or *Knautia* spp. (scabious) and *Tropaeolum majus* (nasturtium). Hoverflies (small wasp lookalikes) will reward the organic gardener with a steady succession of aphid-eating larvae, each of which can gobble up to fifty aphids a day. Bees particularly need sources of pollen and nectar at times of the year when flowers are generally scarce such as early spring and autumn. Aim to encourage them into areas where they are needed for pollination of orchards and other fruit and vegetables.

You should also try to supply some food plants for caterpillars; if there are plentiful supplies of their favourite foods they are less likely to attack your cabbages. A patch of nettles is possibly the best option, but more desirable plants include nasturtium, honesty (*Lunaria annua*), buckthorn (*Rhamnus* spp.), holly (*Ilex aquifolium*), dogwood (*Cornus alba*), ivy and broom. Caterpillars also appreciate thistles, burdock, bramble and wildflowers.

Bee plants

The following are good for providing pollen or nectar:

Acer spp. (MAPLES)
Aster cvs. (MICHAELMAS DAISY)
Berberis spp. (BARBERRY)
Borago officinalis (BORAGE)
Chaenomeles speciosa vars.
  (FLOWERING QUINCE)
Convallaria majalis (LILY-OF-THE-VALLEY)
Cotoneaster cvs.
Crataegus persimilis 'Prunifolia' (THORN)
Crocus spp.
Cytisus spp. (BROOM)
Daphne mezereum (MEZEREON)
Digitalis spp. (FOXGLOVE)
Eryngium spp. (SEA HOLLIES)
Fraxinus excelsior (ASH)
Hedera helix (IVY)
Helenium spp. (SNEEZEWORT)
Hyacinthoides non-scripta (BLUEBELL)
Hyacinthus orientalis (HYACINTH)
Hyssopus officinalis (HYSSOP)
Laurus nobilis (BAY)
Lonicera spp. (HONEYSUCKLE)
Lythrum spp. (LOOSESTRIFE)
Monarda didyma
  (BEE BALM or BERGAMOT)
Nepeta spp. (CATMINT)
Paeonia cvs. (PEONIES)
Phlomis fruticosa (JERUSALEM SAGE)
Potentilla fruticosa
Prunus spp.
  (CHERRY and CHERRY LAUREL)
Pyracantha cvs. (FIRETHORN)
Rhododendron cvs.
Ribes sanguineum (FLOWERING CURRANT)
Rosa pimpinellifolia (ROSE)
Rosmarinus officinalis (ROSEMARY)
Skimmia cvs.
Sorbus spp.
  (MOUNTAIN ASH and WHITEBEAM)
Thymus spp. (THYME)

Tilia x euchlora (LIME)
Ulex europaeus (GORSE)
Verbena spp.

Butterfly plants

Many of the plants that please bees will also attract butterflies. In addition, consider the following:

Achillea millefolium (YARROW)
Agrostemma githago (CORNCOCKLE)
Armeria maritima (THRIFT)
Buddleja davidii, B. x weyeriana and
  others (BUTTERFLY BUSH)
Caryopteris x clandonensis
Ceanothus spp. (CALIFORNIAN LILACS)
Centaurea cyanus (CORNFLOWER)
Centranthus ruber (RED VALERIAN)
Dipsacus fullonum (TEASEL)

Eupatorium cannabinum (HEMP
  AGRIMONY)
Hebe spp. (SHRUBBY VERONICA)
Heliotropium cvs. (HELIOTROPE)
Hesperis matronalis (SWEET ROCKET)
Lavandula cvs. (LAVENDER)
Leucanthemum x superbum
  (SHASTA DAISY)
Phlox spp.
Rubus spp. (BRAMBLES)
Saponaria officinalis (SOAPWORT)
Scabiosa spp. (SCABIOUS)
Sedum spectabile (STONECROP)
Spiraea japonica
Valeriana officinalis (VALERIAN)
Viburnum tinus (LAURUSTINUS)

BELOW Bees are attracted to the rich pollen of *Helenium*, also known as sneezewort!

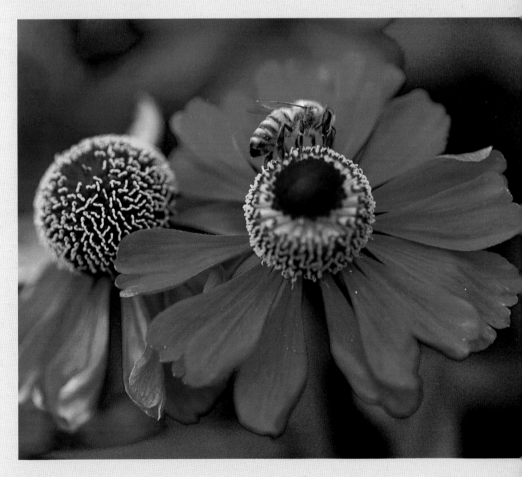

Hedgerows

Hedges are very important habitats for many birds and mammals. Unfortunately they are diminishing daily as they are ripped out by farmers and other landowners. Instead of privet, laurel or the dreaded leylandii, look around to see what grows naturally in your area, or plant a mixed hedge to include any or all of the following:

Acer campestre (FIELD MAPLE)
Cornus sanguinea (DOGWOOD)
Corylus avellana (HAZEL)
Crataegus monogyna (HAWTHORN)
Euonymus europaeus (SPINDLE TREE)
Hippophae rhamnoides (SEA BUCKTHORN)
Ilex aquifolium (HOLLY)
Lonicera periclymenum (HONEYSUCKLE)
Prunus spinosa (BLACKTHORN, SLOE)
Rhamnus frangula (ALDER BUCKTHORN)
Rosa canina (DOG ROSE)
Salix caprea (PUSSY WILLOW)
Sambucus nigra (ELDER)
Viburnum opulus and *V. lantana*
    (GUELDER ROSE and WAYFARING TREE)

Woodland

If you don't have the room to establish a woodland, it is still possible to create a fair imitation of a woodland edge using even a single native tree and a few shrubs (such as those listed above). In the smallest gardens, where every plant needs to justify its space, choose a silver birch (*Betula pendula*) for its elegant bark throughout the year, or maybe even a cultivated version of crab apple (*Malus* cvs.), hawthorn (*Crataegus* cvs.) or rowan (*Sorbus* cvs.), that will have more colourful flowers or berries than its native relative.

Other valuable additions are wildflowers such as foxgloves (*Digitalis purpurea*), which occur naturally in woodland habitats. Ground-cover plants should be chosen from those native to your region; these might include bluebells (*Hyacinthoides non-scripta*), wood anemones (*Anemone nemorosa*) or snowdrops (*Galanthus nivalis*).

Plants for birds

Many birds are excellent hunters of unwanted pests in the garden. Thrushes, robins and blue tits all have a role to play (apart from their individual beauty) as they consume a variety of slugs, snails, caterpillars and other insects.

The provision of water and a variety of proprietary foods in winter will encourage a range of birds into your garden. However, it is equally valuable to provide natural food sources such as seeds and berries, and any plants that offer shelter are worth including. As well as the hedgerow plants listed left, the following are important food sources:

Trees and shrubs

Berberis x stenophylla (BARBERRY)
Cotoneaster spp.
Elaeagnus angustifolia
Hedera helix (IVY)
Malus cvs. (CRAB APPLE)
Prunus padus (BIRD CHERRY)
Pyracantha cvs. (FIRETHORN)
Rosa rugosa (ROSE)
Rubus fruticosus (BRAMBLE)
Sorbus aucuparia (ROWAN)
Symphoricarpos spp. (SNOWBERRY)
Taxus baccata (YEW)

Perennials and annuals

Armeria maritima (THRIFT)
Aster novi-belgii (MICHAELMAS DAISY)
Cosmos spp.
Dipsacus fullonum (TEASEL)
Helianthus annuus (SUNFLOWER)
Iberis spp. (CANDYTUFT)
Lunaria annua (HONESTY)
Oenothera biennis (EVENING PRIMROSE)

RIGHT Foxgloves
brighten up the woodland
habitat, which provides
shelter to a huge variety
of wildlife.

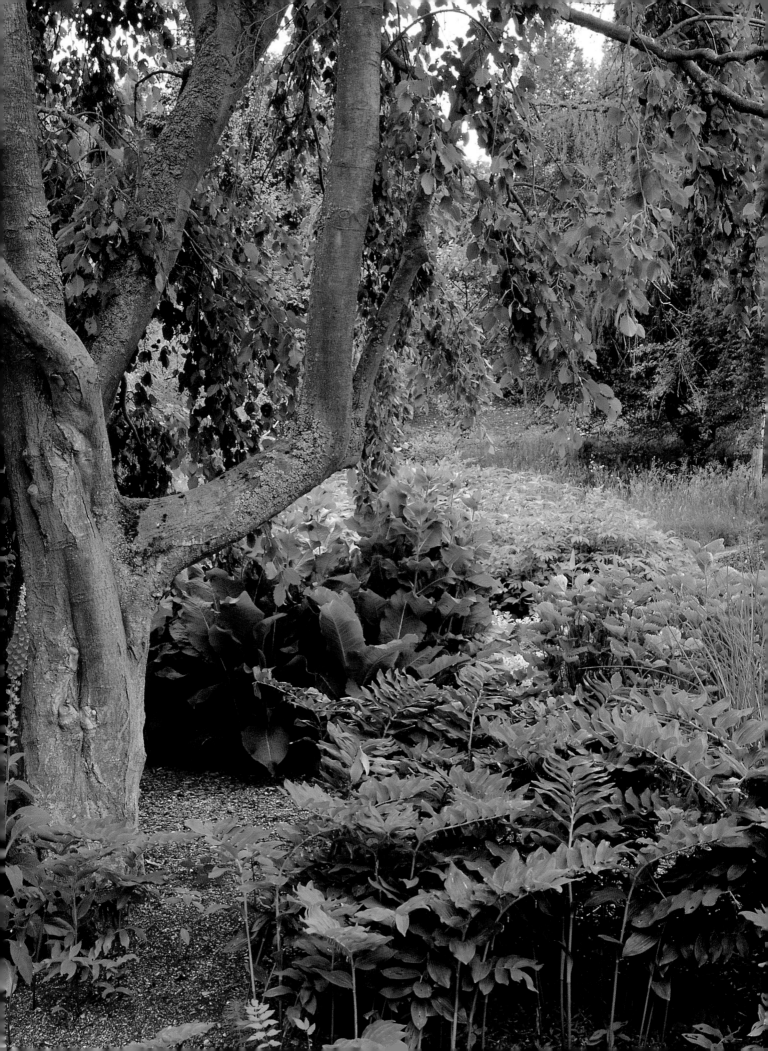

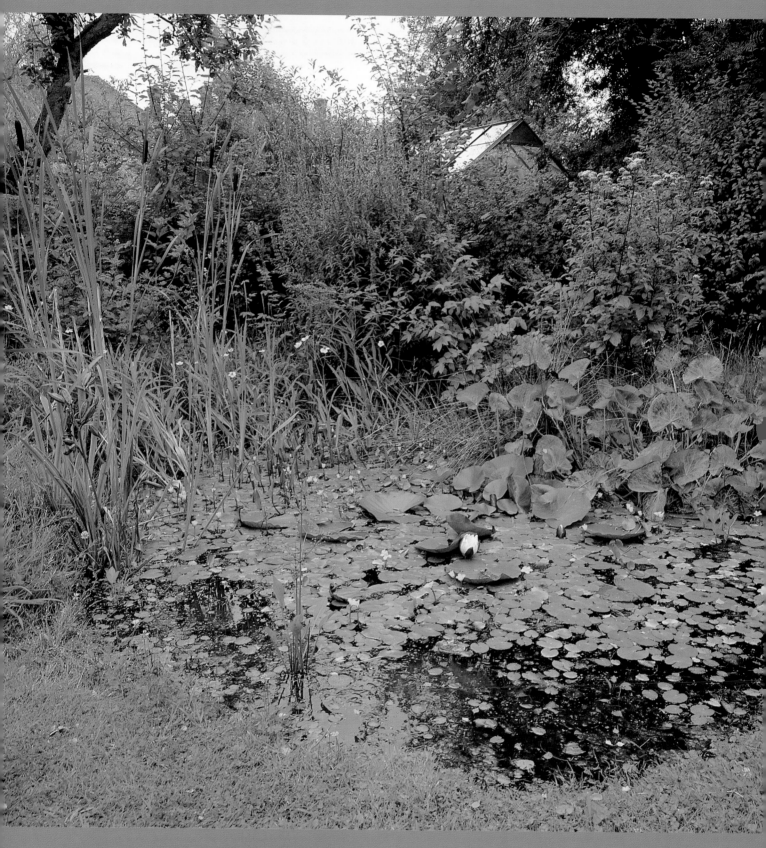

The pond

To create an ideal wildlife habitat in your garden, a pond is a must. Standing water will attract all kinds of animals into the garden, from dragonflies, frogs, toads or newts to birds and mammals such as hedgehogs, which will use it as a bath or watering hole. You will be amazed by what turns up to inspect even the tiniest pond.

Choose a level, open position, away from overhanging trees but sheltered by a backdrop of shrubs and grasses to offer some protection. Aim for a minimum size of 3 metres/8 feet square and, at least at one point, a depth of 75 cm/30 inches. The pond must be easily accessible to animals, so the shallower the gradient of the sides, the better. Depending on your soil, it may be necessary to line the hole with a butyl liner; if so, it is preferable to cover any liner with sifted soil or inverted turves as the finished effect will be more attractive.

A turfed edge will look more natural than stone and will be favoured by visiting wildlife. Fill the pond with rainwater if possible and allow it to settle for a few weeks before putting anything else in. If you have the patience, allow nature to take its course rather than stock the pond with exotic snails or fish, which might cause damage to the native fauna. It is sometimes possible to obtain things like frogspawn from local nature trusts; never remove anything (animal or vegetable) directly from the wild, as many species, such as newts, are protected by law.

Bear in mind that although a wildlife pond is unlikely ever to appear pristine, it will need to be cared for and any dead or over-vigorous vegetation should be removed as soon as possible. Blanket and duck weed should also be kept in check so that the pool does not become entirely choked.

When selecting plants, aim to choose a few from each of the following three sections and pay attention to their likely growth rates to ensure a balance. Stock the pond gradually so that the water surface does not become entirely covered (the shaded surface area should be no more than one third to a half). Native plants are always preferable as they will support the widest range of insects.

LEFT Designed to attract wildlife, this pond is surrounded by bull rushes (*Typha latifolia*), purple loosestrife (*Lythrum salicaria*), meadowsweet (*Filipendula ulmaria*), and hemp agrimony (*Eupatorium cannabinum*).

Oxygenators

These improve oxygen levels and help keep the water fresh and clean. They grow under-water and should be planted directly into the bottom of the pond.

Callitriche stagnalis (COMMON WATER STARWORT)
Hottonia palustris (WATER VIOLET)
Miriophyllum spicatum (SPIKED WATER MILFOIL)
Potamogeton crispus (CURLED PONDWEED)
Ranunculus aquatilis (WATER CROWFOOT)

Deep water aquatics

These grow in deep water with their leaves floating on the surface; they help to shade the water from too much sun. Plant in baskets or directly into soil at the bottom.

Hydrocharis morsus-ranae (FROGBIT)
Nuphar lutea (YELLOW POND LILY)
Nymphaea alba (WHITE WATER LILY)
Polygonum amphibium (AMPHIBIOUS BISTORT)
Sagittaria sagittifolia (ARROWHEAD)

Marginals

These grow at the edge of the pond with their roots directly in water or damp earth. Some will grow equally well in damp soil in a 'bog' garden. Plant in baskets or directly into soil.

Acorus calamus (SWEET FLAG)
Butomus umbellatus (FLOWERING RUSH)
Caltha palustris (MARSH MARIGOLD)
Filipendula ulmaria (MEADOWSWEET)
Geum rivale (WATER AVENS)
Iris pseudacorus (FLAG IRIS)
Lythrum salicaria (PURPLE LOOSESTRIFE)
Mentha aquatica (WATER MINT)
Menyanthes trifoliata (BOG BEAN)
Mimulus guttatus (MONKEY FLOWER)
Myosotis scorpioides (WATER FORGET-ME-NOT)
Scirpus lacustris (COMMON CLUB RUSH)
Typha minima (MINIATURE BULL RUSH)
Veronica beccabunga (BROOKLIME)

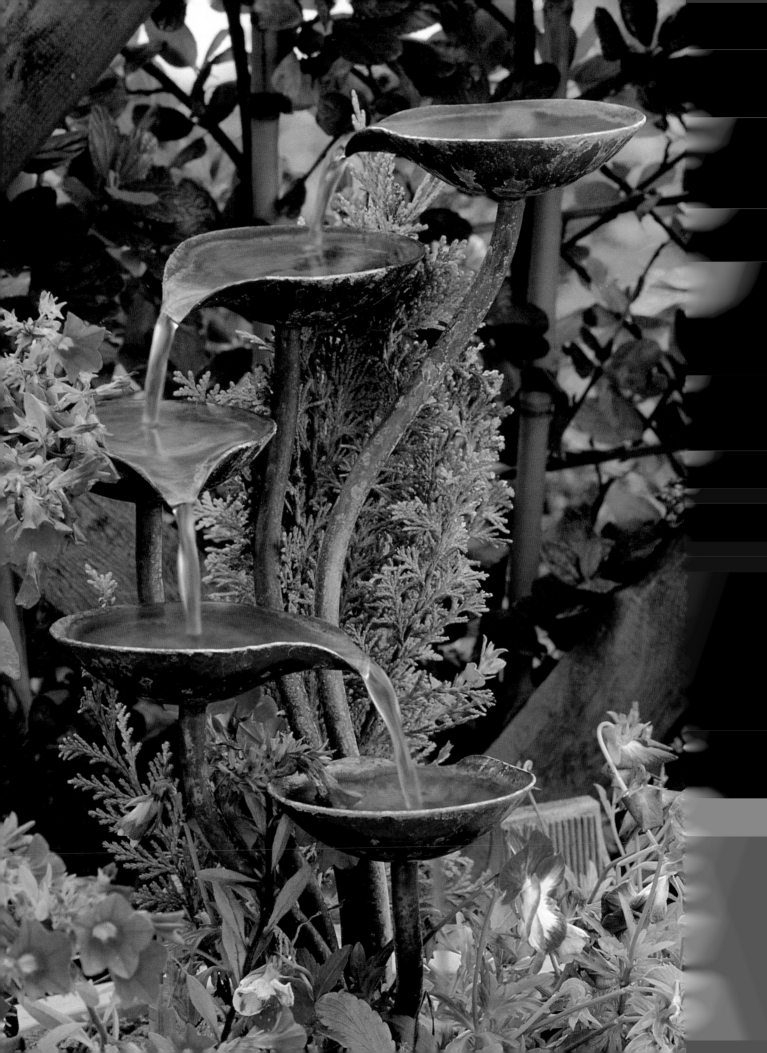

Healthy gardens

Even the most ecologically sound plot can unfortunately be a potential minefield for some people. All gardens have the capacity to generate a multitude of allergens throughout the year, in the form of dust, pollen and fungal spores. These natural triggers can prompt such conditions as hay fever, asthma, skin rashes and other allergies. While many people are susceptible only to certain individual triggers, for others the situation is much more complex and will involve more drastic protectionary measures. Fortunately, there are a number of approaches which can be adopted in order to improve air quality and generally make the garden more 'user-friendly'.

LEFT A cascading water feature acts as an ionizer, freshening the air and improving humidity.

Improving air quality

Clean, fresh air is one of the most valuable resources anyone can have in their garden. An effective way to improve air quality is through a process known as ionization. Ions are gas particles within the air that carry an electrical charge because they have gained or lost an electron. Positive ions are increased by car pollution, cigarette smoke, overcrowding, poor air circulation and the use of synthetic materials. Negative ions are naturally generated by lightning storms and by the breaking of water into small droplets. We often feel uneasy during the build-up to a thunderstorm because of the depletion of negative ions from the atmosphere at that time; lightning then redresses this effect. Plants are also a vital source of negative ions, conducting the earth's negative electrical charge up into the air surrounding them. Coastal areas, bracing upland countryside and inland areas near large bodies of water enjoy a high negative ion content in the air and tend to feel naturally 'healthy' and refreshing.

Ionization cleanses the air through the emission of negative ions, which attach themselves to airborne pollutants and 'ground' themselves to the nearest earthed surface. Increasing the negative ion content of the air around us will therefore clear the air of dust, pollen and smoke, reduce air pollution and so improve overall health. This reduction in dust and pollen levels is of obvious benefit to sufferers of hay fever or asthma. Ideally, the air should contain a negative to positive ion ratio of 60:40. Unfortunately, this is often nowhere near the reality in areas severely affected by everyday pollutants. When positive ions predominate, many people experience headaches, allergies, depression and lethargy (a form of sick building syndrome).

There are a number of ways to redress the balance of negative ions. The use of moving water within a garden is particularly beneficial and fountains or cascades have the combined effect of both freshening the air and improving local humidity. Flowforms are even more potent ionizers; these specially sculptured basins encourage water to flow in a figure-of-eight motion which mimics the movement of naturally flowing water and improves oxygenation.

The growth of lush vegetation will also improve air quality since all plants raise local humidity, cool the air, intercept and 'ground' pollutants, and release oxygen during the day through photosynthesis. In urban areas, plants have a valuable role to play in acting as a barrier to both air and noise pollution. Some plants have been found to be particularly effective at redressing the ion balance; these include ferns, evergreens, palms and ivy.

The circulation of fresh air throughout the garden should be encouraged wherever possible. Try to avoid stagnant areas, which are often caused by impervious windbreaks or excessively dense vegetation. Free air movement will impede the growth of moulds and other plant diseases, leading to a healthier garden all round.

Allergy sufferers may also find the following points worth considering:

- To reduce dust and pollen levels during summer, 'damping down' can be effective – regularly water borders and paving close to the house and around seating areas (if possible, ask a non-allergy-sufferer to do this).
- Good garden husbandry will control fungal growth and minimize the number of spores released in autumn (fungal spores are a common trigger of asthma in some people) – take care to remove all damp rotting vegetation and fruit and keep compost bins well away from regularly used areas of the garden.
- Take care when weeding around or pruning conifers – the needles often act as an irritant and the plants release clouds of dust when agitated.
- Replace hedges with fences; hedges harbour dust and other potential irritants such as spores. Select the timber preservatives you use with care.

- Avoid fruit trees in the garden if anyone in the family has an allergy to insect stings – the rotting fruit will attract wasps and bees.
- Never allow weeds to flower and seed – nettles, docks, mugwort, ragweed and plantain are the worst offenders.
- To keep weeds in check, use gravel as a mulch in preference to bark (which can aggravate allergies caused by dust and fungal spores) and make effective use of ground-cover plants.
- If an allergy to fur means pets are out of bounds, why not consider a fish pond? Water in the garden improves air quality, and fish are very relaxing to watch.

Finally, all allergy sufferers, but in particular those with asthma, need to find a regular and reliable means of relaxation to help overcome the everyday stresses that can so often trigger an attack. To encourage a relaxed body and mind, refer to Chapter 6, Meditation.

Contact allergens

There are a number of common garden plants that are known to cause irritation to the touch. Levels of sensitivity vary and for some people the effects are no more than a minor irritation, but gardeners with sensitive skin or known allergies such as eczema should exclude those varieties which have the potential to cause severe reactions. In many instances, plants have developed a range of strategies to protect themselves from damage. Some species (for example *Fremontodendron*) rely on tiny hairs on the stems to repel predators, while others (for example *Euphorbia*) course with sap that deters even a starving rabbit. It makes sense to take care not to expose bare skin to the following plants, particularly during strong sunlight when reactions are often intensified:

Arum italicum (ARUM LILY) –
   sap can cause skin inflammation
Clematis vitalba (TRAVELLER'S JOY) – irritant sap
Daphne mezereum (MEZEREON) – irritant sap
Dictamnus albus (BURNING BUSH) –
   phototoxic reaction in bright sunlight
Euphorbia spp. (SPURGE) – irritant sap
Fremontodendron californicum –
   minute hairs can irritate skin, nose and eyes
Heracleum mantegazzianum (GIANT HOGWEED) –
   severe phototoxic reaction in bright sunlight
Hedera spp. (IVY) – irritant or may cause allergic
   reaction
Juniperus spp. (JUNIPERS) – needles may be
   irritant
Ruta graveolens (RUE) – phototoxic reaction in
   bright sunlight

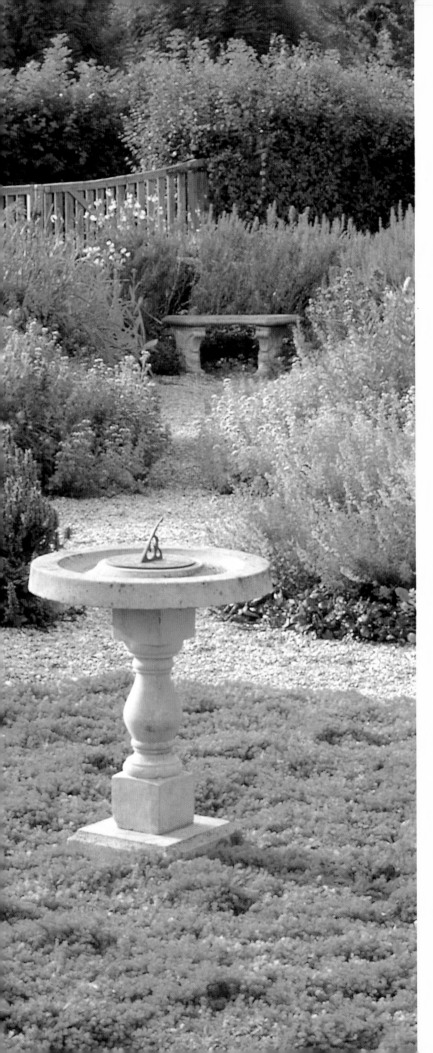

The low-pollen garden

Pollen is one of man's most well-known natural allergens; the body's reaction to it may result in hay fever (a form of allergic rhinitis, where the allergic reaction is in the nose and eyes) or asthma (in which the allergic reaction is in the lungs and airways). Problems can occur at any time of year, but especially spring (tree pollen), early summer (grass pollen) and autumn (weed pollen and fungal spores). Fortunately, most people find they have only very specific sensitivities and if they can discover what triggers the attacks, can do their best to eradicate the source. Although neighbours' plants may thwart your efforts to some extent, the worst offenders can at least be eliminated from your own garden. Through careful selection of species, floating pollen levels can be reduced considerably.

Most grasses – including ornamental varieties such as *Cortaderia selloana*, *Festuca glauca* and *Stipa gigantea* – are a huge source of pollen when in flower, and it is therefore sensible to avoid a lawn altogether or at least keep it to a minimum size (and encourage someone else to mow it regularly without ever allowing it to flower). If the alternatives of paving or gravel are unacceptable, why not consider a small lawn of perhaps thyme or chamomile – although harder to establish, the end results are very rewarding. Ensure you use only lawn chamomile, a non-flowering variety called 'Treneague' or you will simply be adding to your problems!

Other wind-pollinated plants, which release pollen to be carried by air, should also be avoided. These mostly carry their flowers as catkins and tend to be trees, although there are also a few shrubs worth excluding:

Acer spp. (MAPLES)
Alnus spp. (ALDER)

LEFT Chamomile makes a fragrant alternative to a grass lawn and will be enjoyed by all, including hay-fever sufferers.

Betula spp. (BIRCH)

Carpinus spp. (HORNBEAM)

Corylus spp. (HAZEL)

Fagus spp. (BEECH)

Fraxinus spp. (ASH)

Garrya elliptica

Itea ilicifolia

Platanus spp. (PLANE)

Populus spp. (POPLAR)

Quercus spp. (OAK)

Salix spp. (WILLOW)

Ulmus spp. (ELM)

A few conifers can also cause allergies through their light pollen:

Chamaecyparis spp. (FALSE CYPRESS)

Cryptomeria japonica (JAPANESE RED CEDAR)

Cupressus spp. (CYPRESS)

Juniperus spp. (JUNIPERS)

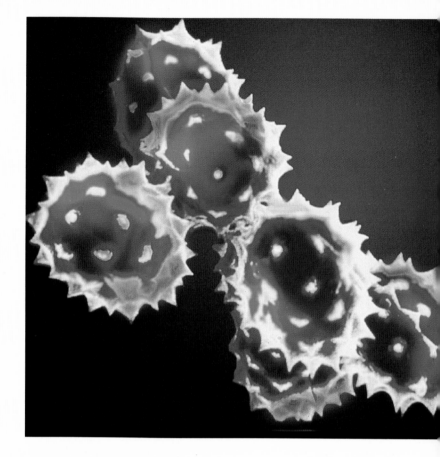

Other particularly allergenic plants are members of the families Caryophyllaceae (pinks) and Compositae (daisies and thistles, which have recently been reclassified as Asteraceae). Plants from these families are likely to produce some of the worst reactions in allergy sufferers.

Besides carnations and pinks (*Dianthus* spp.), the Caryophyllaceae family includes such popular border flowers as *Gypsophila* spp. (baby's breath), *Lychnis* spp. and *Saponaria* spp. (soapworts).

The Compositae family includes many common garden plants, but don't despair – a little research should enable you to find suitable alternatives. Some seasonal annuals may also give rise to problems if planted en masse and should therefore be avoided; these include dahlias, marigolds and osteospermums.

Achillea spp. (YARROW)

Anthemis spp. (CHAMOMILES)

Artemisia spp. (WORMWOOD)

Aster spp. (MICHAELMAS DAISY)

Centaurea spp. (KNAPWEED)

Chrysanthemum spp.

Coreopsis spp. (TICKSEED)

Cynara cardunculus (CARDOON)

Echinacea spp. (CONEFLOWER)

Echinops spp. (GLOBE THISTLE)

Eupatorium spp.

Gaillardia spp. (BLANKET FLOWER)

Helenium spp. (SNEEZEWORT)

Helianthus spp. (SUNFLOWERS)

Helichrysum spp.

Inula spp.

Leucanthemum vulgare (OXEYE DAISY)

Liatris spp. (GAY FEATHERS)

Ligularia spp.

Olearia spp. (DAISY BUSH)

Rudbeckia spp. (CONEFLOWER)

Santolina spp. (COTTON LAVENDER)

Senecio spp.

Solidago spp. (GOLDEN ROD)

Although it may limit others' enjoyment of your garden, it is also wise to avoid highly scented flowers, as strong perfumes may trigger allergic reactions in some people:

Jasminum officinale (JASMINE)

Lilium cvs. (LILIES)

Philadelphus cvs. (MOCK ORANGE BLOSSOM)

Strongly scented roses

ABOVE A cluster of pollen grains from a member of the daisy family, seen under an electron micrograph.

Good plants for a low-pollen garden

Insect-pollinated plants, which rely on bees and winged insects for pollination, produce heavier, stickier pollen which is less likely to be carried on the wind and therefore inhaled. There are many suitable garden varieties, including any of the following:

Amelanchier spp. (SNOWY MESPILUS)

Berberis spp. (BARBERRY)

Buddleja davidii (BUTTERFLY BUSH)

Ceanothus spp. (CALIFORNIAN LILAC)

Choisya ternata (MEXICAN ORANGE BLOSSOM)

Clematis spp.

Cornus alba (DOGWOOD)

Cotoneaster spp.

Crataegus spp. (HAWTHORN)

Euonymus fortunei

Fuchsia spp.

Geranium spp. (CRANESBILL)

Hebe spp. (SHRUBBY VERONICA)

Hosta spp. (PLANTAIN LILY)

Iris spp.

Lavandula spp. (LAVENDER)

Magnolia spp.

Malus spp. (CRAB APPLE)

Paeonia spp. (PEONY)

Phormium tenax (NEW ZEALAND FLAX)

Photinia 'Red Robin'

Picea pungens (SPRUCE)

Potentilla fruticosa

Prunus spp. (FLOWERING CHERRY)

Robinia pseudoacacia (FALSE ACACIA)

Salvia officinalis (SAGE)

Spiraea spp.

Viburnum spp.

There are also many plants which, through various strategies, have evolved to produce little or no pollen. Some plants produce mostly sterile flowers and release minimal amounts of pollen:

Bergenia cvs. (ELEPHANTS' EARS)

Hydrangea anomala subsp. *petiolaris* and many other lacecap hydrangeas

Phormium cvs. (NEW ZEALAND FLAX)

Polemonium spp. (JACOB'S LADDER)

Viburnum opulus 'Sterile' (SNOWBALL TREE)

Vinca minor (LESSER PERIWINKLE)

Most plants with double flowers, where the stamens have been modified to form extra petals, are sterile. Some of these varieties are brought about by natural mutation while others have been bred and selected by nurserymen for larger, longer-lasting flowers:

Caltha palustris 'Plena' (MARSH MARIGOLD)

Clematis 'Vyvyan Pennell'

Houttuynia cordata 'Flore Pleno'

Paeonia lactiflora 'Duchesse de Nemours' and P. 'Sarah Bernhardt' (DOUBLE PEONIES)

Prunus avium 'Plena' (GEAN)

Some plants have naturally sticky or hairy leaves which trap and hold pollen and dust, thus reducing free levels within the air:

Alchemilla mollis (LADY'S MANTLE)

Clematis cvs.

Convolvulus cneorum

Heuchera cvs.

Hydrangea aspera subsp. *sargentiana*

Phlomis fruticosa (JERUSALEM SAGE)

Pulmonaria cvs. (LUNGWORT)

Salvia argentea

Stachys byzantina (LAMB'S EARS)

For fragrance in the garden, allergy sufferers would be wise to select plants which provide scent through their leaves, although a few people may even have a reaction to the essential oils produced by certain herbs (for more information refer to Chapter 5, Aromatherapy): Many herbs are suitable, including lavender, rosemary and sage.

Choisya ternata (MEXICAN ORANGE BLOSSOM)

Cistus spp. (ROCK ROSE)

Eucalyptus spp. (GUM TREE)

Houttuynia cordata

Phlomis fruticosa (JERUSALEM SAGE)

Rosa rubiginosa (SWEET BRIAR)

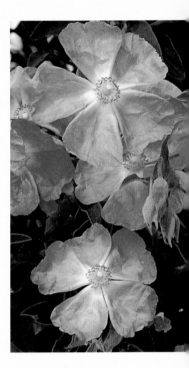

ABOVE *Cistus* 'Peggy Sammons' is insect-pollinated and flowers freely in early summer.
BELOW *Hosta* 'Big Daddy' for low-allergy ground cover.

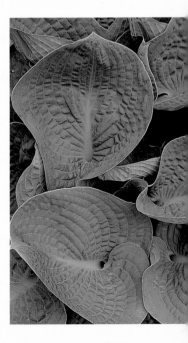

The edible garden

For many, a garden is not complete unless it contains a few plants that are grown for the sole purpose of being eaten. One of the greatest joys of gardening is sending your taste buds into raptures over the flavour of 'real' fruit or vegetables. Growing your own produce is the only way to capture the true essence of strawberries, tomatoes or even peaches, which need to be eaten straight from the plant. Freshness will never be in doubt and you will be able to grow unusual crops which might not be available from your local shop. Last, but not least, if you garden organically, you can also be sure that your produce is free from harmful residues.

In our eternal quest for convenience, the seasons have gradually blurred into a year where strawberries are available at Christmas and satsumas can be bought throughout the summer. Although this provides us with more choice than ever before, most supermarket produce is a mere facsimile of its former self, often devoid of taste and scent. There is something reassuring about picking and eating apples when they are supposed to be harvested, and enjoying tomatoes that have ripened in the sun instead of on a shop shelf.

If you want to rediscover such simple pleasures, there is no need for a kitchen garden spanning many acres. Most seed suppliers have now fully embraced the concept of 'mini-vegetables' which are ideally suited to the smallest plot. Almost any vegetable can be successfully grown in a container and there are even trailing tomato varieties that are designed to grow in hanging baskets! However, there is one restriction – don't grow food crops near busy roads or in inner city areas which may be badly affected by air pollution.

Every garden will have room for a few plants, even if these are simply pot-grown strawberries or a single miniature fruit tree. Don't ignore spaces between other plants in a border; many vegetables now come in colourful varieties and are ornamental in their own right, for example ruby chard (see page 71), oakleaf lettuce, purple podded beans or the ferny fronds of asparagus. Vegetables grown among other plants will have the benefit of companion planting (see page 18) and small pockets of plants are less likely to be picked out by the pests in the first place. Another method to prevent the build-up of pests and diseases is regular crop rotation – never grow a vegetable in the same spot for more than one season.

The easiest and fastest plants to raise are undoubtedly salad vegetables. Lettuces, spring onions and radishes have a very short cropping time and can even be grown in a few orange crates if there is no other space in the garden. First make a list of your personal favourites and then consider the room you have in your garden – it is surprising how many varieties can be grown with a little careful planning. So-called catch crops, where fast-growing plants such as lettuce are grown between slower varieties, can effectively double your available space.

It is possible to grow fruit in most gardens. A larger area will support a range of soft fruit (strawberries, raspberries, blackcurrants, red-currants) and top fruit (apples, pears, plums, cherries, peaches). You may even set aside a segregated space, perhaps an orchard or a fruit cage. However, many varieties will thrive in a small garden if their selection and cultivation is matched to their allotted area.

Strawberries can be grown very successfully in pots and a container will even support a gooseberry or blackcurrant bush. These might be trained as standards to introduce a formal element and free the ground beneath for further planting. A thornless blackberry or tayberry can be trained across a trellis or over an arch, where it takes up very little space. It is also possible to grow fruit trees in containers if suitable varieties are grafted on to dwarfing rootstock and the plants are kept well watered and fed. Where space is limited, choose either self-fertile varieties or plant a 'family' tree to ensure successful pollination. In the latter, branches of one or two other varieties are grafted on to the original tree – for example a Cox's Pippin apple tree could have a branch bearing Golden Delicious and another bearing Bramleys.

Many varieties of apple, pear and cherry can be grown successfully as fans, cordons or espaliers against a fence or wall. These make very effective living 'screens' which might be used instead of trellis.

Finally, herbs are a valuable feature in any garden. If there is enough space, a separate herb garden could be built (see Chapter 4, Herbalism), but many herbs are ideally suited to growth in pots. Those of Mediterranean origin such as sage, rosemary and thyme actually prefer the improved drainage in containers, while others, for example mint, are best kept restrained to curb their rampant tendencies!

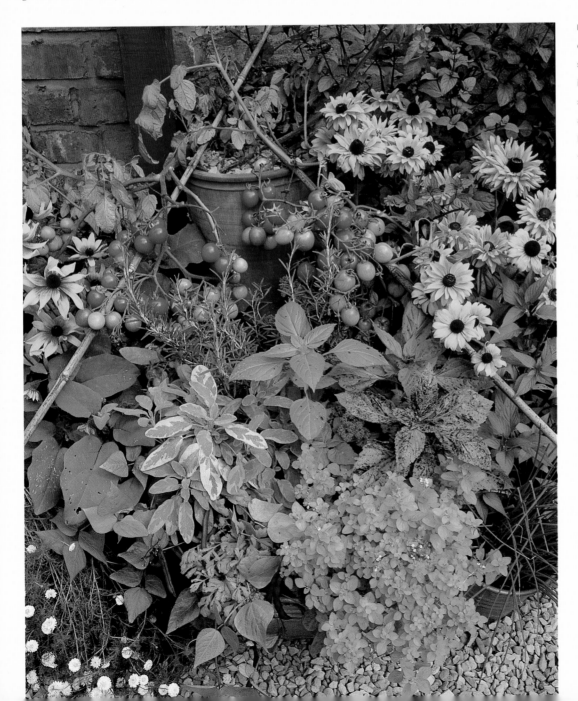

LEFT It's amazing what can be grown in a small space: this planting includes basil, variegated sage, golden marjoram and rosemary with French bean 'Purple Teepee' and tomato 'Tumbler' trained along canes. Even more colour is provided by the rudbeckia, which looks perfectly at home in the company of its unusual bedfellows.

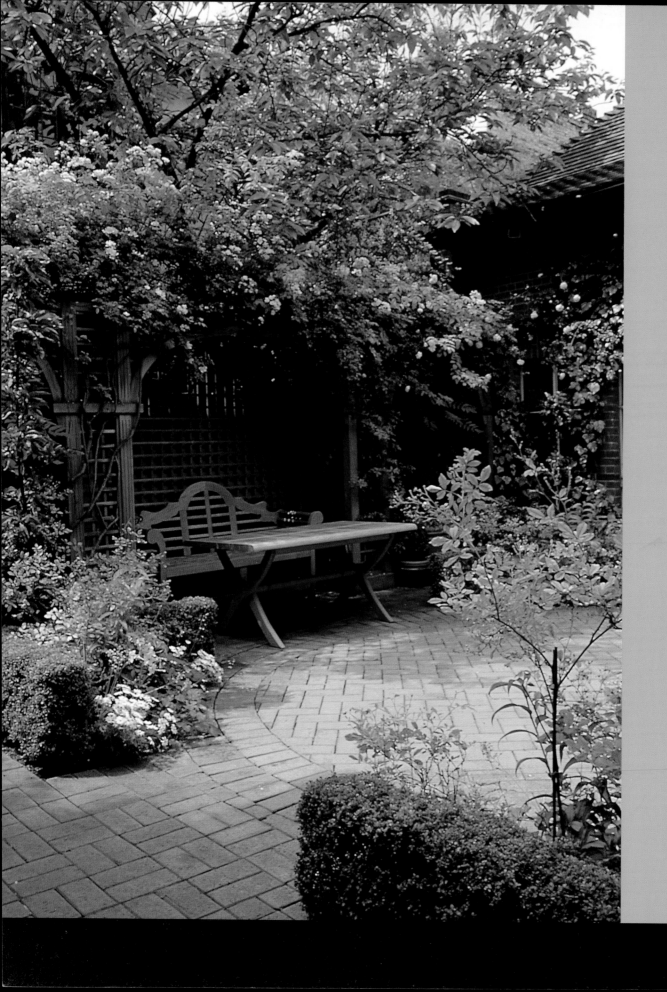

2

Feng shui

There is no logical way to the discovery of these elemental laws. There is only the way of intuition, which is helped by a feeling for the order lying behind appearance.

ALBERT EINSTEIN

Feng shui is many things to many people. Some know it as an ancient Chinese practice based upon folklore, while others see a more scientific side. In a spiritual sense, *feng shui* is rooted in Taoism, a religion whose followers acknowledge the power of nature and seek to live in harmony with it. However, *feng shui* can also be seen as a creative and intuitive philosophy which blends common sense with prudent design to create a more balanced environment.

Feng shui has evolved through the meticulous observation and analysis of human interaction with our environment. The practice has developed into a system of holistic design that studies the way in which our surroundings affect our well-being, happiness and success. There is currently widespread acceptance that the location and arrangement of our homes not only reflects our lives but can also shape them; either supporting us or, conversely, bringing about misfortune. These concepts seem ever more relevant and can be related to topical problems such as global warming, sick building syndrome and overhead power lines.

Feng shui differentiates between auspicious and inauspicious sites; those with 'good' energy being sought for their beneficial influences over every aspect of life. 'Bad' sites are avoided as they have the potential to bring about disasters including illness, divorce or financial loss. A practical function of *feng shui* is the specific arrangement of your immediate environment in order to improve your life fortunes through an awareness of, and alignment with, the earth's energy lines. This invisible energy, referred to as *ch'i* or *qi*, is present throughout the universe in all living things and inanimate objects and it can be detected and utilized for healing. The *feng shui* master may use a special compass, or *luo pan*, to indicate the potential of both beneficial and harmful influences. *Feng shui* also takes account of topography, psychology and astrology, some of which may be seen as superstition in the West. Its serious study involves an apprenticeship which can take many decades to complete. A single chapter cannot do this vast subject justice; it is intended simply as an introduction.

Feng shui may involve strange new concepts but it also has much to do with common sense. Quite simply, we need to change the way we look at things and learn to live in harmony, rather than in conflict, with the natural world. If you remain unconvinced of your own abilities, you might wish to invite a professional to give you a personal reading; helpful addresses can be found on page 168.

LEFT *Ch'i* (invisible energy) is continually flowing around us throughout our everyday surroundings. This garden, open in the centre (the *tai ch'i*) allows the healthy movement of *ch'i*. The area also appears balanced in terms of light and shade, formal and informal planting and the ratio of planting to paving.

Feng shui principles

Ch'i or qi

Ch'i is a term used to describe the life force of the entire universe. Everything around us, in the earth, water and heavens, has an 'energy' with the potential to affect us. We can now control light, sound and electricity, but there are other types of energy that we have not yet learnt to measure. *Feng shui*, literally 'wind and water', symbolizes two such energies.

The primary aim of *feng shui* is to tap into the beneficial qualities of *ch'i* and use the forces of nature to create a healthy, balanced flow of energy in your immediate environment. For a site to be auspicious, it needs characteristics which themselves promote a sense of health, harmony, beauty and comfort. In a garden, rich, fertile land, with gently rounded features and a balance of plant form, colour and texture will represent good or *sheng ch'i*. Unkempt landscapes with rough or sharp features represent negative or *sha ch'i*. *Sha ch'i* is a destructive force which is naturally present in cold winds, still, dank air, stagnant water and poorly drained soil. Fault lines in the earth's crust may also produce *sha ch'i*, as do fast roads or rivers, power cables, tunnels, railways and drains.

Yin and yang

The terms *yin* and *yang* are used to describe the fundamental dualism of natural forces; together, they constitute 'the way' or *Tao* – the principle of universal harmony whose life and breath is *ch'i*. Everything in the universe contains both *yin* and *yang* energy in varying proportions. Without one, the other cannot exist and each contains within it a seed of its opposite (represented by dots in the *tai ch'i* symbol). In simple terms, for light to exist there must also be dark and there can be no heat without cold. The entire universe is thus composed of opposites, some of which are listed here:

Yang	Yin
hot	cold
light	dark
day	night
noise	quiet
dry	wet
active	passive
high	low
hard	soft
sun	rain
male	female

Through their opposing qualities, a flow is created which forms a never-ending cycle of change, a natural rhythm which produces and embraces every aspect of life. As the two energies ebb and flow, day and night each take turn and a seasonal cycle is created where *yin* energy rules winter, *yang* governs summer and the two are balanced at the spring and autumn equinoxes. When the two energies exist in harmony, good fortune is produced; any imbalance will manifest as misfortune.

Every aspect of our surroundings may be categorized according to its essential nature. Rivers, roads, mountains, hills and buildings all create *yin* or *yang* energy which affect the *feng shui* of a place. Windy hills or mountains and fast-flowing water are described as *yang*, whereas *yin* energy is greatest in valleys or low-lying areas and near still pools or gentle streams. The most auspicious landscapes are those where *yang* and *yin* are in harmony, with gently undulating features and containing a balance of rock, water, vegetation and open space.

The five elements

Ch'i is believed to manifest itself both actually and symbolically through five elements: water, fire, wood, metal and earth. These fundamental archetypes of life energy are to be found in our everyday surroundings. In creating a harmonious environment, the aim is to look for missing elements and, at the same time, ensure none is overly dominant: the ideal is to strive for a balance between all five. Initially this may seem hard to achieve, but symbolism plays a vital role here, elemental shapes being found in every aspect of our surroundings. Colour also provides clues to the identification of the energies. Ground conditions are often excellent indicators of the dominant element: boggy ground equates to water; barren, rocky landscapes to fire; and forested areas to wood.

● Water

SEASON: winter
COLOURS: black, dark blue
SHAPES: wavy or horizontal

Typical garden features: ponds, fountains and streams or *yin* objects (gentle colours, soft forms)

● Fire

SEASON: summer
COLOUR: red
SHAPE: triangular

Typical garden features: flowers in warm colours such as red, paving with angular patterns, light, heat (barbecues or candles) or *yang* objects (strong colours and forms)

● Wood

SEASON: spring
COLOUR: green
SHAPES: rectangular, tall, straight

Typical garden features: trees, upright plants, green foliage, timber posts, wooden features

● Metal

SEASON: autumn
COLOURS: white, gold, silver
SHAPES: curved, domed

Typical garden features: metallic or rounded stone ornaments, white or light-coloured stone paving

● Earth

SEASON: early autumn
COLOURS: yellow, brown, orange
SHAPE: square

Typical garden features: ceramic or terracotta pots and ornaments, clay pavers, bare earth, earthy colours

Energy cycles

Rather as *yin* and *yang* or night and day continually flow into each other, the energies of the five elements interact with each other in both creative/supportive and controlling cycles.

Consideration of the cycles is necessary to ensure that any features in your garden will be mutually beneficial and harmonious. If one element is too weak, it can be reinforced by adding its supportive element or removing its controlling element – or vice versa. For instance, in summer, as plant growth in the garden becomes dominant and threatens to overwhelm its surroundings, the addition of water will add to the problem, as water creates wood (represented by green foliage). On the other hand, the introduction of metal (or stone) into the area will help to redress the balance as metal controls wood. This could also be taken literally – metal shears could be used to trim back plant growth.

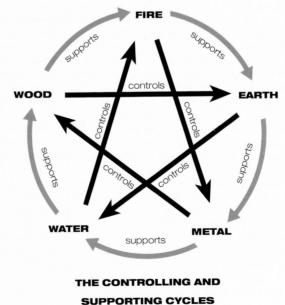

**THE CONTROLLING AND
SUPPORTING CYCLES**

The compass school

When rigorously applied, this technique uses computations based on the eight trigrams (Chinese characters) of the *I Ching*, the directions of the compass, planetary influences, the five elements and an individual's date of birth; it incorporates a combination of metaphysical speculation, symbolic association and complex calculation. With these inputs, the *feng shui* of a place is interpreted through precise placement of the *pa kua* symbol, the *lo shu* square (the magic square, an ancient numerological device) and the Chinese compass or *luo pan*.

According to the compass school, every sector has a different energy and any house, room or garden may be divided into eight distinct areas (nine including the centre). Each represents a key aspect of life, such as relationships, wealth, health, education or career. Fortune can thus be enhanced by making improvements to the appropriate area(s), either strengthening the basic energy type or reducing its force by adding a controlling element (see previous page). A compass is required to identify the sectors. The area relating specifically to health will lie within the eastern sector of the garden, but the centre is also considered important.

The *pa kua* can be extended in any direction to fit houses and gardens of all shapes, but always remains square, rectangular or octagonal in outline. If the area being considered does not form a regular shape, any missing sections are deemed to be 'missing space'. This can have an impact upon the related area of your life (see page 56 for further information on how to counter this).

Pa kua

The *pa kua* (sometimes spelt *ba gua*) is an octagonal symbol from which is derived the ancient philosophical oracle, the *I Ching* or *The Book of Changes*. The concept of the *pa kua* is deemed to have a powerful influence over everything in the universe, and forms the basis of the compass school of *feng shui*. Each of the eight trigrams around the edges of the *pa kua* is made up of three lines which symbolize heaven, earth and humanity; the lines may be broken (*yin*) or unbroken (*yang*). Each trigram has a symbolic meaning (closely allied to the energies of the five elements) and corresponds to points of the compass, numbers, colours, members of the family, parts of the body, emotions and spiritual qualities and other aspects of life. Through careful interpretation, the *pa kua* enables the study of the particular attributes of any section of a house or garden.

South

Recognition/fame

Fire

9

Associations: red, purple, lights, personal achievement, midsummer

Southeast

Wealth/prosperity

Wood

4

Associations: green, bright blue, planting and small trees, the compost heap, early summer

Southwest

Relationships/marriage

Earth

2

Associations: yellow, orange, groups or pairs of plants or features, a wilder, informal style, late summer

East

Family/health

Wood

3

Associations: green, tall plants or trees, a potting/growing area, spring

The Tai Ch'i (unity)

Health/spirituality

5

The central area should be uncluttered, clean and orderly. It might include water (only if always clean, fresh and moving)

West

Children/creativity

Metal

7

Associations: silver, gold, white, metallic objects, a children's play area, autumn

Northeast

Education

Earth

8

Associations: yellow, orange, blue, an area for relaxation, a cultivated/formal area, late winter

North

Career

Water

1

Associations: black, dark blue, water (ponds, fish, waterfalls), a clear, open area, midwinter

Northwest

Helpful people/Mentors

Metal

6

Associations: silver, gold, white, metallic objects, meditation, wildlife areas, late autumn

The landscape or form school

This school of *feng shui* predates the compass school approach and requires a close study of your surroundings in order to interpret the symbolism of the landscape. The natural world pulses with invisible energies which are considered either auspicious or inauspicious. Clues are present in the shape and location of hills, rocks, buildings, water courses, roads, hedges and trees. Although it originated from the study of the rural landscape, it can be adapted to the urban environment. In this instance, awareness switches to power lines, flyovers, bridges, railways, telegraph wires, drains, neighbouring houses and pylons.

For *feng shui* purposes, the perfect location (in the northern hemisphere) is an open, south-facing slope, protected by hills to the north with a stream to the front. A view of water to the front, such as a pond, lake or the sea is also auspicious. From a practical point of view, these descriptions make a good deal of sense as a house that faces south will obviously be bathed in warm sunlight for most of the day. Such a location also has the best chance of benefiting from a healthy balance of elements: good air quality with both gentle wind and moisture, workable soil, a mixture of light and shade and pleasant views. A house at the top of a hill is exposed to all the elements and may be lashed by wind and rain from every direction; conversely a house at the foot of a hill is at risk of flooding during heavy storms.

Water has a vital role to play, signifying wealth and fertility and being an excellent source of *ch'i*, but only when clean and gently flowing. Stagnant, polluted or dirty water should be avoided at all costs as it represents negative energy or *sha ch'i*, which will lead to ill health. The ideal situation is to be embraced by a gently meandering stream or river, with no sharp turns. If it is in the wrong place or of an undesirable shape, water can create serious health problems. A view of water is preferable to actually living near it; this applies particularly to the sea, which is impossible to control and therefore potentially dangerous. Practical reasons for not living too near water are the detrimental effect it may have

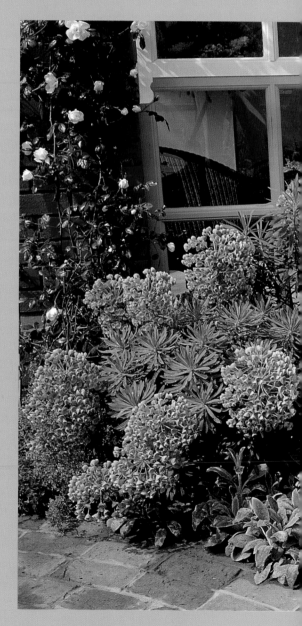

upon the foundations of a house and upon health, damp air being associated with breathing difficulties and joint problems.

Practising feng shui

These days, many practitioners choose to combine the two schools, although 'landscape' factors will always override compass calculations as they are physically more powerful. This is especially true if any particularly harmful influences are found through the landscape method; these must not be ignored since it is practically impossible to mitigate them through management with the compass method alone. A great deal can be achieved through symbolism, but some people may find the need for intuitive insight of the landscape system difficult to implement. Although the compass system may be harder to grasp initially, it does become easier to practise. Since there is relatively little most of us can do about the actual location and surroundings of our home (in the short term at least), this chapter will concentrate on the compass school approach.

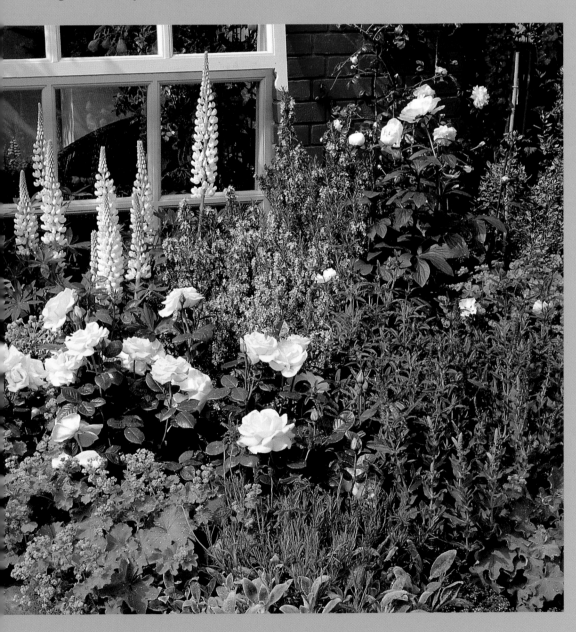

RIGHT Although a beautiful composition in terms of colour, texture and form, the plants in this border are beginning to grow above the windowsill. They will soon block both views out and the free passage of *ch'i* into the room, which may lead to stagnant energy in that sector of the home. Either plant low-growing species at the outset or be prepared for an annual pruning session to keep the plants in check.

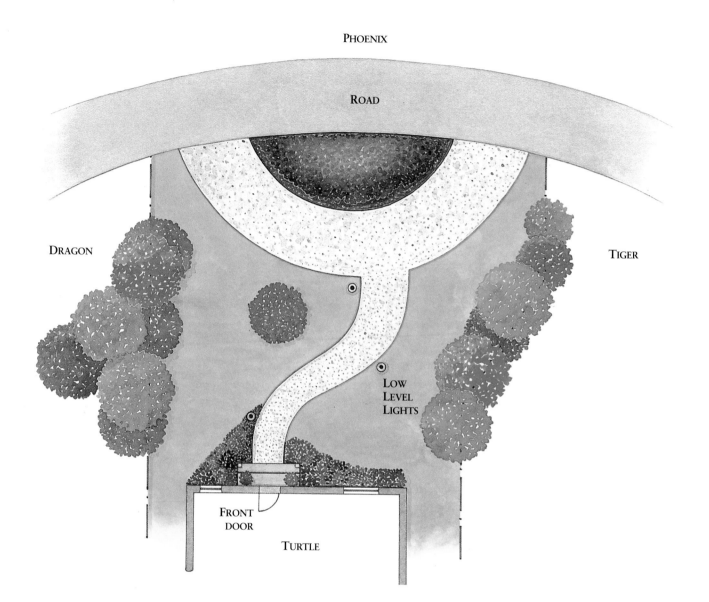

PHOENIX

ROAD

DRAGON

TIGER

LOW
LEVEL
LIGHTS

FRONT
DOOR

TURTLE

Landscape principles in an ideal front garden

The plot is generally level, and planting towards the front (phoenix) is kept low, to allow views out. Lighting maintains a sense of openness at night. Small trees or tall plants protect and defend the right-hand (tiger) side; planting to the left (dragon) should be taller. Don't forget that neighbouring gardens should be included in your survey. On either side of the front door are containers planted with healthy evergreens and perhaps seasonal annuals. Borders in front of the house include a mixture of low-growing plants which provide colour, texture and form throughout the year. The curve of the drive deflects *sha ch'i* which may emanate from the road, and a carefully placed small tree protects the front door from possible poison arrows. The meandering path regulates the flow of *ch'i* into the house.

Celestial animals

The concept of four celestial animals is used to portray *feng shui* requirements through symbolism. Any location – for example your bed or work desk – may be considered in relation to the celestial animals in order to discover whether it is auspicious or not. Referring more specifically to the garden, the following directions are taken looking out of your front door:

● Green dragon – to the left

The 'dragon' is symbolized by a hill, house or tree(s) which should not be as high as the 'turtle' to the rear of the house but taller than the 'tiger' to the right. It represents wisdom and the need to look ahead.

● White tiger – to the right

This should be a hill, tree(s) or house, lower than the one to the left; the 'tiger' should never be larger than the 'dragon' or misfortune will be brought upon the occupants of the home. It represents physical strength and can both defend and attack. Since it has the capacity for violence, it needs to be controlled.

● Black turtle – to the rear

The 'turtle' is symbolized by hills behind the house which protect it from attack and cold winds and represent support and security. Such protection is also afforded by taller houses or trees. A site should never have a drop to the rear as this exposes the occupants to danger. Large bodies of water at the back, such as a river or lake, are generally considered undesirable, and can lead to health problems.

● Red phoenix – to the front

This should be a low-lying, open area, which may be enhanced by a small hillock to symbolize a footstool (indicating a comfortable life). It represents the ability to look far ahead; the 'phoenix' passes information to the 'dragon'. It is considered very inauspicious to live in a house with a hill or steep slope upwards immediately in front of its main door; a plot in a gentle depression is acceptable as long as there are views out.

Adjusting your surroundings

It is obviously very rare to find the perfect site according to all the *feng shui* principles. However, the fundamental concepts are relatively easy to seek out in any landscape. Where desirable elements are missing, the imagination comes into play and adjustments can be made either physically or symbolically in order to encourage a healthy circulation of *ch'i*.

Many Western homes lack a large front garden or perhaps face undesirable barriers or hills to the front, while benefiting from a gently sloping rear garden with good views. In this instance, although surrounding topography and the architectural facade of the house must be taken into account, it may be advisable to reverse the directions and consider the rear garden as your front ('phoenix') and the front garden as the 'turtle'. In this way, energy in the important area outside your front or main door can be maintained as open and circulating, which will encourage healthy *feng shui*.

Poison arrows

All practitioners of *feng shui* recognize the potential dangers of unfavourable *ch'i* or *sha ch'i*. This may come from stagnant energy, caused by clutter, neglect, dust and damp, or from *ch'i* energy moving so quickly that it could easily get out of control, destabilizing those in its path. A particular type of *sha ch'i* is often termed the 'poison arrow' or cutting *ch'i*. It could be compared to the point of a knife, and has the effect of disturbing the flow of *ch'i*, leading to ill health. 'Poison arrows' act as channels for inauspicious energy and are harmful if aimed at any part of a plot, but particularly at front doors or areas where you spend a lot of time.

Sha ch'i arises from straight, sharp-angled or pointed lines within the landscape and it is vital to recognize these lines in order to deflect detrimental energy. Almost any object or structure can create *sha ch'i*; in addition to straight lines, it also emanates directly out from the right-angled corners of features such as walls, ponds and paving. If you are able to design your garden from scratch, take great care when using strong geometric shapes such as squares and triangles; better perhaps to incorporate informal curves or circular designs.

Of course, trees, roads and other straight lines feature in many situations, but there are a number of steps that can be taken to mitigate their effect (for further ideas, see page 52):

- wind chimes can be hung to calm the flow of fast-moving *ch'i*
- straight lines within your garden can be softened by planting over their edges (see page 53)
- straight lines or sharp angles directed at your property can be screened from view by planting a hedge or shrub between them and your plot
- a mirror, shiny letterbox or even a coat of glossy paint could deflect cutting *ch'i*

Any of the following may constitute a 'poison arrow' and should be avoided (or remedied) wherever possible:

- any sharp, angled or pointed object either directed at, or in close proximity to, the main door
- electricity pylons, power stations or lines, railway tracks, telegraph poles, flyovers or bridges
- any object with a threatening appearance
- you should also be aware of shadows cast on to your property by anything straight

Roads

- houses on the outside of a bend or facing a sharp corner
- a plot facing a T junction or a dead end
- houses situated around a roundabout
- any fast, straight roads

Neighbouring houses

- corners of neighbouring houses or rooflines which point at your house
- a narrow gap between two opposite buildings (block from view if possible)

Water

- houses where a river or bridge points directly at them
- sharp bends in water courses and fast-flowing water in a straight line

Plants

- tall, narrow trees or a single tree trunk immediately outside a door or window
- plants with sword-shaped leaves in close proximity to a path or seating area

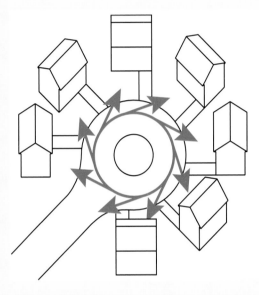

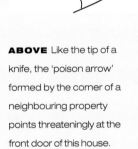

ABOVE Energy spins off a roundabout as a constant series of 'poison arrows', which might affect every house in this cul-de-sac.

BELOW The house inside the bend is safe from the energy of the road; the other two are at risk from *sha ch'i* travelling in straight lines.

ABOVE Like the tip of a knife, the 'poison arrow' formed by the corner of a neighbouring property points threateningly at the front door of this house.

BELOW The fast-flowing *ch'i* directed straight at the house by this T junction puts it constantly 'under attack' from uncontrolled energy.

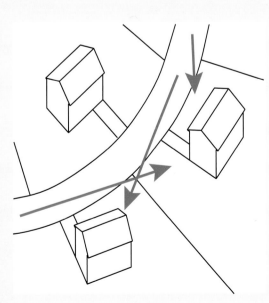

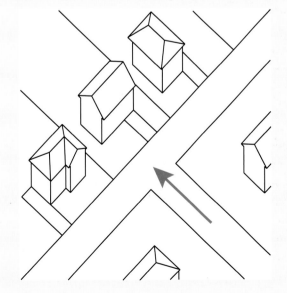

Feng shui in the garden

RIGHT The timber
decking, green-blue
wood stain and lush
vegetation of this garden
relate to the east, the
sector of the *pa kua* most
closely related to health.
Any of these elements in
the eastern area of your
garden will activate wood
energy and have a
beneficial effect upon
your health. Beware,
though, of overdoing any
such 'cure': this area is
lacking the balance of
other elements such as
fire, metal and earth,
which may be detrimental
in the long run. The
addition of some warmer
colours would counter
the excess *yin* qualities
and create a more
balanced arrangement.

Although in existence for thousands of years in the East, many people in the West have encountered *feng shui* only recently. A few will have applied simple techniques to their home, but much of the available information has concentrated on interiors and has not been widely adapted for use outside. However, the same theories apply and can be successfully translated to the garden to bring about improvements to health and well-being.

The practice of *feng shui* requires a very individual approach and consequently every garden should reflect the characteristics and personal situation of its owners. At the same time, no matter what its size or location, the planning and layout of a garden is normally dictated by accepted design guidelines. This section will deal with the integration of *feng shui* into the garden as a whole and is intended to encourage an open mind in order to assess potential problems.

The plot

Whether you are looking at a new house with a view to moving, or simply reconsidering your existing one, the immediate surroundings play an important part in the *feng shui* of a place. Take a little time to look closely at what surrounds you.

If you are considering moving into a new development, exposed land is considered to have unstable earth *ch'i* and damage should be remedied by appropriate planting as quickly as possible. It is advisable to avoid houses near areas that are still being developed and to allow some time for the land to settle before moving in.

The most auspicious plot shape is regular with parallel sides. If there is a particularly weak side, or a corner of the plot has been cut off, it constitutes a 'missing space' and might create difficulties in your life (this could be countered by following some of the advice on page 56). A triangular plot is very inauspicious and a house built on such a plot, where the front of the house actually faces the point, will cause the occupants to suffer from ill health. Jutting edges or corners, which might create cutting *ch'i* (see previous page), should be rounded off wherever possible or may be camouflaged with trees or plants grown on the boundary.

The scale of the house should be in proportion to its setting. If it seems overpowering, make an attempt to 'enlarge' the garden visually, by retaining more open space and using outdoor lights, smaller plants and lower fences. The placement of your home within the plot warrants some attention; if you are building your own home, you may even be able to dictate its precise location. The provision of adequate space around the house is important and the dwelling should be sited fairly centrally. Aim to give a well-defined area to the garden so that it is not simply cramped into the spaces left over from the house.

The boundaries should preferably follow natural features such as contours, streams or hedgelines, but gardens are more commonly marked by either a wall or fence. In such cases, neither should be so close to the house that it gives a feeling of being trapped; ideally, any barrier should be at least two metres from the house. Boundary fences and walls should be blended into the landscape wherever possible so that they protect the house and garden but do not

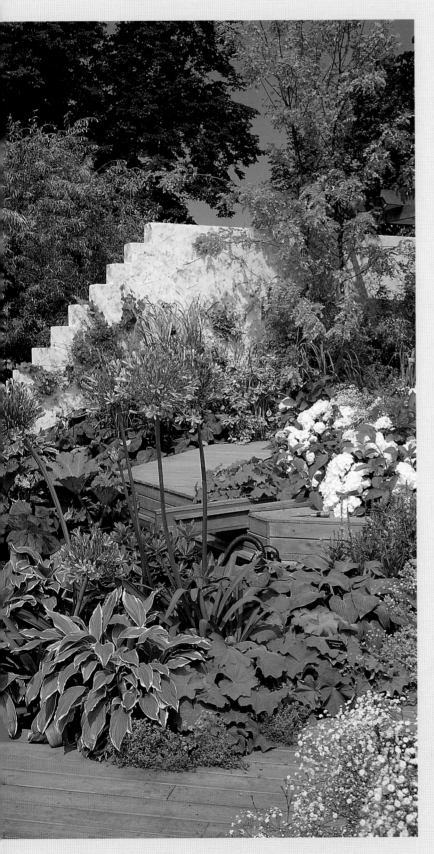

overpower them. If your boundary seems too straight or rigid, the effect can be softened by placing a border of plants in front of it. Spikes and arrows on fences should not point down because this implies descent in life; nor should they point inwards as these create cutting *ch'i*.

Ground conditions are also important, the ideal soil being well aerated and neither too wet nor dry. Although this situation is desirable it is obviously not always possible to achieve, but bear in mind that the soil type, if particularly wet or arid, may have a detrimental effect upon you, not just the plants in your garden. Soil can be improved by the addition of organic compost, which will help dry soil to retain moisture and promote drainage of wet soil.

The house exterior

Harmony may be achieved through a property that merges with its surroundings. Colour can counteract excess *yin* or *yang*, for instance using strong, bright (*yang*) colours to combat excessively *yin* features.

The house shape should also be considered in order to avoid the 'missing space' of 'L' or 'U' shaped houses, which can lead to misfortunes in the relevant area(s) of your life. Always give a great deal of thought to the size and position of any proposed extension or garage to ensure you don't detrimentally affect the existing balance of a house. For similar reasons, avoid houses with too many awkward corners, which create 'poison arrows'. Houses containing courtyards are, however, considered auspicious because an element of nature can be contained at the centre of the house (*tai ch'i*).

Ideally, there should be a step up into the house; this is because roads are equated with rivers in that they invite danger if you are below their level. The step(s) should be stable and solid and if there are a number of steps, they should be wider at the bottom, narrower towards the top.

A garden which slopes or steps up from the front door may cause problems and a door which opens on to a solid wall or similar obstruction is equally inauspicious as either will block the free flow of *ch'i* into the home. The door should ideally open on to a clear, flat path without interference from any structures. The area immediately outside the door should be well lit at night and kept clear of rubbish and dead leaves and any clutter such as log stores, bins or wellington boots.

The front door to your home is its most important feature since most *ch'i* energy enters the house through it. The door is particularly at risk from 'poison arrows' (see page 48), which must be remedied immediately they are discovered. Since plants produce beneficial *ch'i*, you could place planters containing evergreens (for good health) and flowers on either side of the front door. The plants must, however, be kept living and healthy at all times.

Drives and front gardens

The drive is a major pathway of *ch'i* from the road to a house; its layout and materials should be aesthetically pleasing and in keeping with the style of the house. A circular or semi-circular driveway is preferable, ideally with a meandering approach to control the flow of energy. Avoid at all costs a drive that heads straight for the front door; where a straight drive is unavoidable, the edges should be softened with plants to break up and camouflage the hard lines.

Level and in proportion to the building, the drive should be neither too narrow nor wide. If possible, it should be slightly wider at the entrance and taper toward the house; this applies equally to any path to the front door. Particularly wide driveways encourage the loss of *ch'i*, especially if they slope downhill. In this instance, lamps at the front door will help to control the flow. However, tall lamp posts must never be placed directly outside the front door because they create cutting *ch'i* and block the inward flow of *ch'i*. Blown light bulbs should be replaced immediately.

Any path to the front door should meander gently, avoiding straight lines. If it cannot be curved, use a well-placed pond, small tree or shrub to deflect *sha ch'i* travelling straight between the road and the front door. Heavy items such as boulders, concrete balls or statues placed on either side of the front gate or door

are auspicious, but choose them with care to suit the scale and character of your house. They will prevent *ch'i* escaping and protect the house, while more ferocious stone figures such as lions will help to deter burglars.

The front gate should ideally be made from metal with a soft, curved design and, like the front door, it ought to open smoothly, silently and easily.

Plan your front garden to require minimal maintenance so that it appears welcoming and attractive at all times. To reduce the time spent mowing tiny patches of grass in an urban garden, gravel is often a suitable alternative, which will suppress the growth of weeds. A balance of elements is auspicious: a pond or fountain, a carefully selected and positioned tree, mixed flower beds, an element of stone in the form of a statue or boulders, and an outdoor light will bring varied energies to the area.

Garden design and features

When planning your garden, the primary aim is to shape the energies of the garden by using a balance of the various elements. Make use of natural, local materials wherever possible to harmonize your home with its environment, and remember to look beyond your own boundaries at the surrounding influences.

A harmony between *yin* and *yang* is simply achieved through the creation of both bright, warm areas which encourage activity (*yang*) and shady, quiet places for gentle contemplation (*yin*), as well as a balance between soft (planting) and hard landscaping (building materials). Incorporation of the five elements will further enhance *feng shui* and might involve the juxtaposition of boulders in ground cover planting, plants breaking through gravel, vertical tree trunks set against rounded hillocks, the incorporation of streams, ponds, or waterfalls, and a harmony of colour and light.

In order to encourage the gentle and continual circulation of healthy *ch'i* within the garden, straight lines should be avoided. Although the central area of the garden should be kept relatively clear, 'barriers' such as trellis or plant borders may be incorporated

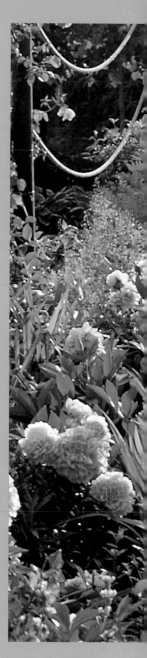

BELOW The inauspicious nature of a straight brick path is defused by the lush planting on either side, which billows over the edge and gives the illusion of a meandering route.

towards the perimeter to prevent a through flow of energy. Paths should be curved and kept towards the edges of the garden; keep them clear of bins, rubbish and overhanging plants at all times so that the energy can move freely around.

Any garden features such as ponds, gazebos or summerhouses are best based upon a rounded shape as curves do not emanate cutting *ch'i*; even more auspicious is the *pa kua* shape (an octagon).

Some variation in the levels will prevent monotony within the garden and, although a flat site is acceptable, a totally contourless garden will be improved by the addition of plants, ponds, boulders or trees to create variations in height. If carefully planned, changes in level can also help contribute to the 'celestial animals' philosophy (see page 47). A raised rear garden, or elevated hillocks to the rear of the house, will improve the 'turtle' aspect, and if the

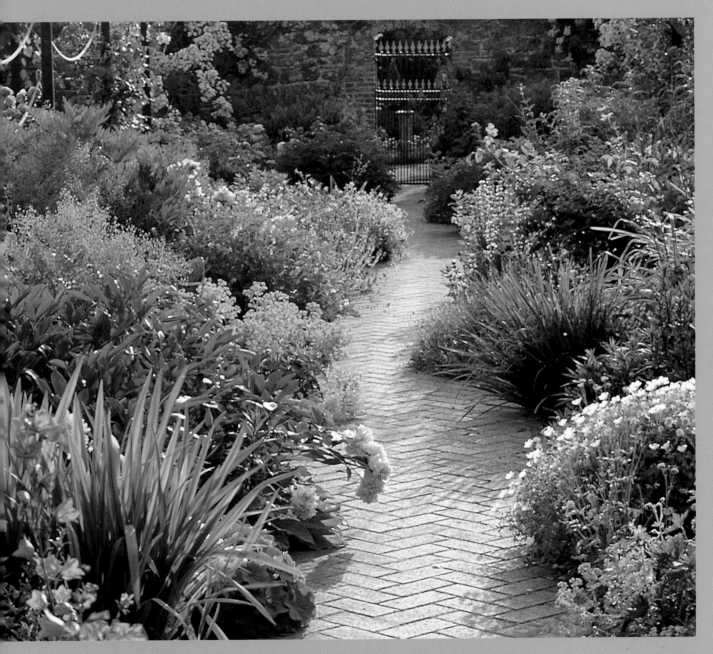

RIGHT An arbour such as this creates a sheltered and private spot for a couple to relax and enjoy each other's company. The muted tones of the plants and scent of the roses will encourage a sense of romance. The pair of dogs act as a guard against unwanted intrusions.

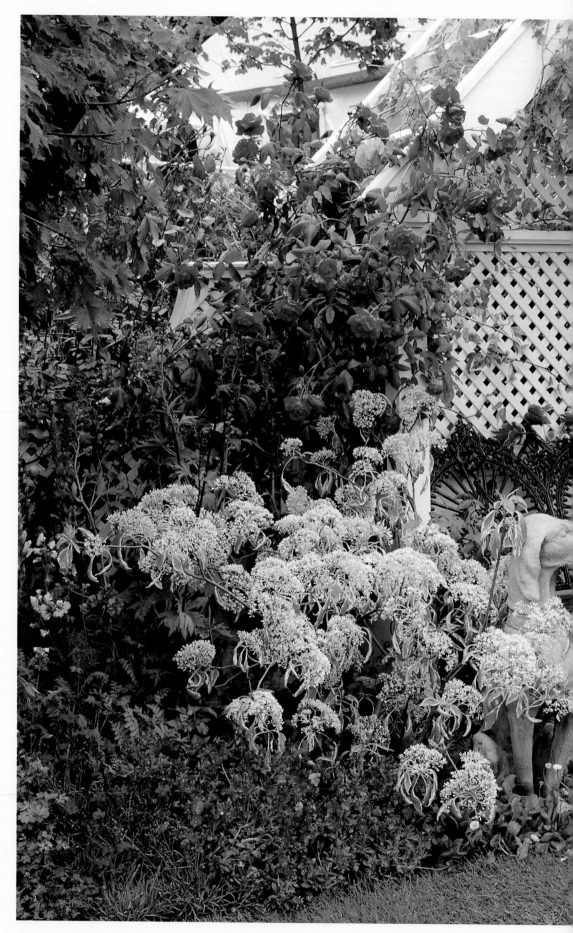

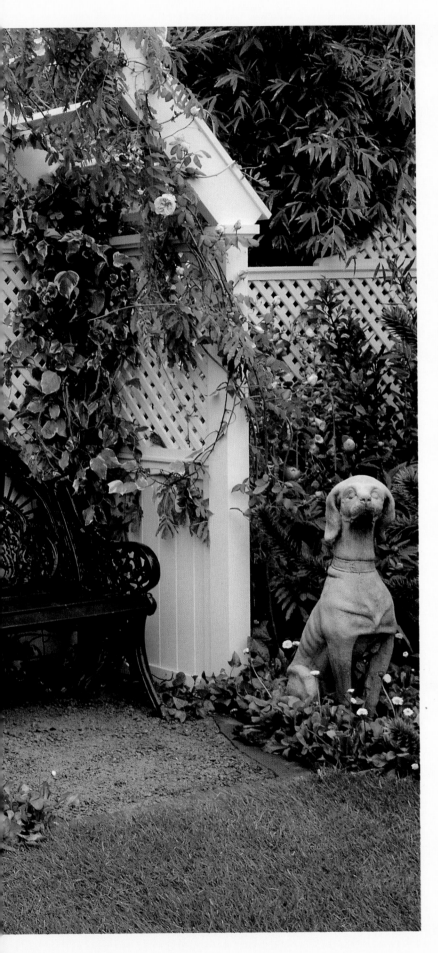

garden itself is contoured in any way, the highest point should be on the 'dragon' side.

Where space allows, aim to divide the garden into distinct areas so that it is not all visible in one glance but gradually entices you from one space into another. You might provide a section for children with bright colours, a sandpit, swings or a den; an area for you and your partner with a secluded seat surrounded by soft, romantic colours, fragrant flowers and a pair of statues to keep the partnership stable; a quiet, contemplative place for yourself with a water feature and a gazebo or summerhouse, screened from the remainder of the garden.

Sculpture within the garden can be very beneficial, especially when its symbolism is used to 'activate' a particular area. Always choose pieces with soft contours and avoid hard angles. To achieve balance in all things, cultivate some of the garden and leave the remainder to grow more naturally so that there is a harmony between formality and informality, man and nature. This approach will also have the benefit of encouraging wildlife into the garden, which is considered to be very auspicious. In addition, frogs and other aquatic dwellers will help to keep any water clean and healthy.

The seasons have an important influence over the garden, governing different tasks at different times. Spring requires a clear-out, symbolizing the start of a new cycle; it is also an auspicious time to make any changes to the garden. Summer is full of *yang* energy and needs areas of shade and cool, restful places to offset the heat and riotous colours. Autumn demands another clean-up and the removal of dead and dying plants. Winter is a time to add warm, bright colours to counter the *yin* energy and balance the cold. Learn to recognize the subtle shifts within the garden which are brought about by the changing seasons and celebrate the passing of time with suitable activities.

Feng shui for health

Many people now accept that an holistic approach is important for good health. In *feng shui* terms, overall health is not just about feeling well but also enjoying happy relationships and success in all aspects of your life – which can be brought about if your home contains beneficial *ch'i* energy in every area. This section focuses on specific measures that might be adopted in the garden with the aim of creating a space that is both beneficial to health and aesthetically pleasing.

In order to make a difference, it is necessary first to consider any problems in your life (particularly recurring ones) and try to relate them to the present state of your surroundings, then make any necessary adjustments. You need to be clear about your objectives before you begin, and only when you are fully aware of the environment in which you live can its energies be activated or sedated in order to effect the remedy you are hoping to achieve. A detailed *feng shui* evaluation of a garden can be quite complex, especially when it is part of a mental or physical healing process. If you have serious issues to address, the support of an experienced *feng shui* consultant is highly recommended.

Tackling problems

Most difficulties can be counterbalanced with harmonizing treatments, but the type and scale of the problem will have a bearing on the remedy. The element of time also needs to be considered; for instance, if trees are required as part of a 'cure', they will take some time to grow to a suitable size and other steps may need to be taken in the interim.

As we have seen, *feng shui* seeks to increase the flow of positive energy and subdue the negative in order to create harmony throughout the environment. To do this, both a reactive and proactive stance may be required, switching between defence and enhancement tactics as necessary. In basic terms, this means deflecting *sha ch'i* and

encouraging *sheng ch'i* by ensuring a balance between *yin* and *yang* and the five elements.

Begin by taking an overview of the garden, using the guidelines in the previous section. Next, clean out all clutter so that you can clearly see your present situation – this is simply a matter of removing all dead plants and rubbish, exposing the 'bones' of the garden and perhaps giving the pond, if you have one, a proper clean.

A vital step is to check for sources of *sha ch'i* such as 'poison arrows', and remedy them wherever possible in order to defend against any harmful influences (see previous section). The most important issue is the protection of your front (or main) door. In the short term, a *pa kua* (octagonal) mirror (or any other small convex mirror) may be hung outside the door to deflect *sha*. The garden can also be specifically designed to protect the plot or house from direct views of roads, lamp posts or other such problems, placing large plants, trees or other features between yourself and the source in order to disperse *sha ch'i*.

'Missing space'

Another important aspect is that of 'missing space'; if an area is missing from the outline of your house or garden, this could have a detrimental effect, and it is necessary to take action in order to avoid misfortune. Where the area is missing from the house shape, fill it in wherever possible in order to complete a square or rectangular outline. This might be achieved with an extension or conservatory, or a patio laid so that the area appears linked to the house rather than the garden. If your plot is an irregular shape, could the missing area(s) of land be bought to make it symmetrical?

If none of these are feasible, there are other techniques to activate the missing energy of that area and create balance. One is to locate a pond or birdbath within the space missing from the house so

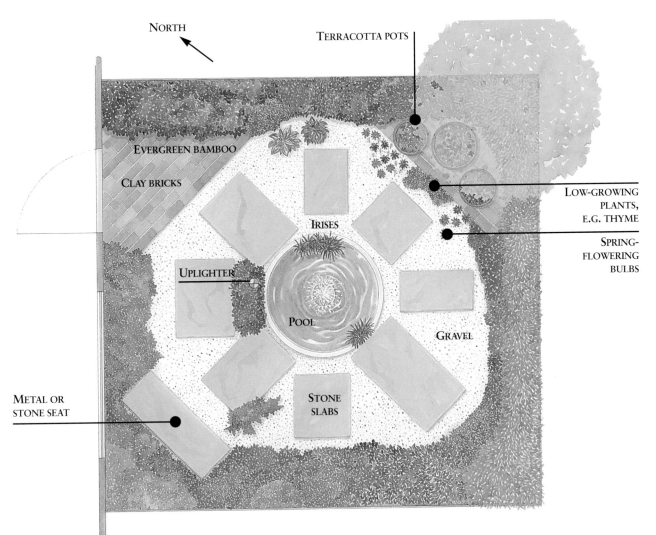

NORTH

TERRACOTTA POTS

EVERGREEN BAMBOO

CLAY BRICKS

IRISES

UPLIGHTER

POOL

GRAVEL

LOW-GROWING
PLANTS,
E.G. THYME

SPRING-
FLOWERING
BULBS

METAL OR
STONE SEAT

STONE
SLABS

A small garden for optimum health

This layout would be suitable on a terrace or roof garden. The pool brings beneficial *ch'i* to the centre (*tai ch'i*), but it is important that it is kept clean and that its size does not dominate its surroundings. A fountain would be a valuable addition and an uplighter to illuminate the water will enhance its healing effect. Although water is supportive of wood, ensure it is not overpowering; the upright growth of the irises around the pool will counterbalance the *yin* of the water. Any plants, but particularly a small upright tree, in the eastern sector will bring wood energy to activate *ch'i* for health. Early-flowering bulbs such as crocus associate with spring (the season related to wood) and the number three might be represented by pots. Take care that other elements are not overwhelmed: a metal or stone seat in the western corner will help with this.

that the water will activate the missing energy; it must, however, be well maintained and clean. A bright lamp, positioned in the far (imaginary) corner of the 'missing space', will flood the area with light and appear to bring it back into the *pa kua*.

Mirrors may also be used to give the illusion of an area where it does not in fact exist. They can reflect another part of the garden into that sector of the *pa kua* that is missing. Used to reflect a specific 'cure' such as a water feature, plant or statue, a mirror will 'double' its effect and can therefore produce a very potent energy.

Activating positive energy

Once these protective steps have been taken and harmful effects mitigated as far as possible you can then attempt to 'activate' the *ch'i* within your garden. The basis of the compass school relies upon this 'activation' of the different sectors of the *pa kua*, which relate to the eight life aspirations. The garden is divided into eight spaces with an additional central area. When the *pa kua* is superimposed on a plan of the garden, each sector's characteristics can be identified and individually considered. The issue of health is most related to the east and the *tai ch'i* (centre) of the garden, but overall health is also associated with your surroundings as a whole and so the state of your entire garden is important.

For a specific health problem, it is advisable to contact a *feng shui* practitioner (as well as a doctor), as individual parts of the body are governed by specific elements connected to the time of our birth.

In order to achieve harmony between the elements, first look at the existing garden to see if any element is overpowering and, if so, aim to enlarge the remaining ones (actually or symbolically) or introduce another to counteract this imbalance. For example, if a terrace seems to be all stone, soften it with billowing planting along its edges and through cracks in the paving; if a seat feels too hard, add some cushions; and if your garden is overhung by trees, cut them back to let light through. Remember at all times that a sense of scale is of paramount importance.

There are, however, no hard and fast rules in this application of *feng shui*, simply a need for creative solutions to problems. Much of the subject is a matter of personal interpretation and cures will need to be tailored to individual requirements. In general, if something makes you feel good, stick with it.

Carry out changes one at a time and allow at least one month for the results to show, since time is

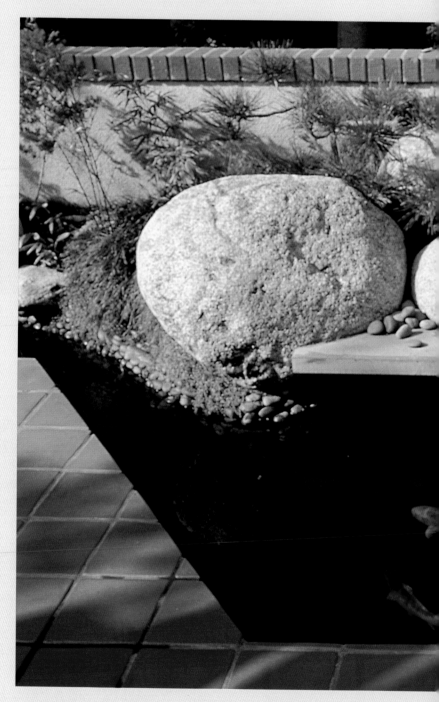

required for the beneficial *ch'i* to enter and harmonize your life. Always act slowly and gradually so that you have time to evaluate any differences before you move on to the next alteration. Carefully consider the scale of any items in an area so that you use a cure of an appropriate size and make sure you don't overdo it. Enhancers or 'cures' which are commonly employed to bring about beneficial changes are as follows:

Water

Water is full of positive energy; it cleanses and revitalizes its surroundings, attracts wildlife and enhances health if well positioned. However, any

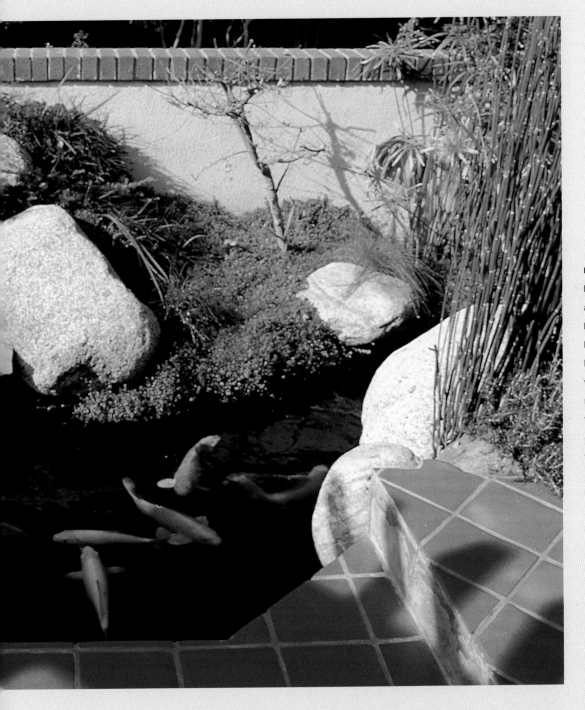

LEFT A small pond can be tucked into any appropriate corner to bring auspicious energy – but the water must be kept crystal clear and the whole area well maintained. Several tactics can be adopted to ensure the *yin* energy of the water is not too overpowering, especially if positioned near the house. The water is balanced by the wood of the surrounding plants, and the metal energy of the boulders; it is countered particularly by the fiery *yang* nature of the red tiles. The seven fish will further offset the *yin* characteristics.

water within the garden must be carefully sited and kept scrupulously clean. Decaying plants must be removed immediately as they produce *sha ch'i*.

Water can be used to neutralize an overpowering fire energy. It has a powerful 'cooling' effect upon the atmosphere and will make a sun-baked corner feel more comfortable. Moving water will activate the energy of any area; fountains, waterfalls and streams all have slightly different influences. The upward, revitalizing motion of a fountain is to be preferred as the downward energy of waterfalls can equate to loss of wealth, unless counterbalanced by a pool beneath of an appropriate size.

The living energy of fish is also highly beneficial and will double the beneficial power of water. Goldfish or koi carp help energize the flow of *ch'i* and further enhance success and prosperity, particularly when placed near the entrance to the home. They should be kept in odd numbers, which are *yang*, to offset the *yin* of the water. Dead fish must be removed and replaced immediately or their *yin* presence will be overpowering.

The most auspicious shape for a pond is round or octagonal – the shape of the *pa kua*. Failing this, informal shapes with curved sides are also suitable; the corners of square or rectangular shapes should at least be rounded off. The style of the pool should blend with the character of the house and the size should be in proportion with its surroundings; the nearer to the house, the smaller it should be. Birdbaths are useful in small gardens, but must be kept clean. The most beneficial position for a pond is outside the main entrance to the home, where it will enhance general good fortune.

The presence of water to the rear of a house is believed to lead to missed opportunities. It is also said that if there is a pond at both the front and back of a house, young children will find survival difficult. The reasoning behind this is, surely, self-evident! Ponds should therefore generally be avoided in the back garden, although there are instances where this landscape school advice might be reversed (see page 47). However, since water has such an important role to play in garden design, water in the back garden

can be countered with the following measures. Keep the pond well away from the house and use *yang* plants, such as those with upward growth and bright flowers, to re-establish a balance. *Yin* plants such as those with a drooping or cascading habit and softly coloured flowers should be avoided around a pond.

Swimming pools also conflict with the rule of avoiding water to the rear of the house. If you choose to have a pool, it must be set well back from the house and should never be larger than the house itself. An informal, curved shape is preferable and straight edges or geometric shapes should be avoided.

Open drains and gullies should always be covered with a suitable filter to prevent soil or leaves clogging them and restricting the removal of dirty water. Manholes should be disguised wherever possible, using recessed manhole covers, or covering them with pots of plants to prevent *ch'i* being flushed away and to counteract the *sha* which emanates from them.

Plants

Plants bring an auspicious energy and stimulate activity in any area of the *pa kua*, but they associate particularly well with the health-related eastern area, since their 'wood' energy is beneficial there. Almost all plants will encourage *ch'i* in the garden; the larger and healthier the plant, the more *ch'i* is generated. There is only one proviso – the plants within your garden must be kept healthy at all times, since diseased or dying plants can signify and cause ill health. Always remove dead, dying or diseased plants immediately to negate their *yin* energy; regular deadheading is recommended for the same reason.

Trees and other large plants can help to provide the symbolism of the 'celestial animals' and may be used in place of hills or buildings to create a more auspicious location. Planting toward the left ('dragon') boundary should be taller than that on the right ('tiger') side. A clump of trees, particularly evergreens, can be used to give 'turtle' protection where no other shelter exists. The 'phoenix' aspect (front) should be kept relatively clear so that open views are retained. The central area of the garden should also be kept clear.

Trees and large plants can also be used to deflect 'poison arrows' caused by sharp corners, acute angles and straight paths. Trees produce powerful fields of energy and are potent transformers of *sha*, thus acting as protectors of a site. Evergreens are considered especially beneficial (except when placed in the south) because their leaves produce *ch'i* continually throughout the year. However, if a tree is unhealthy in any way, it will have the opposite effect, draining life energy away. It is therefore vitally important to treat all trees with the respect they deserve and care for them if they become unhealthy or damaged. If badly diseased or scarred, they should be removed at once. Such problems are very often a sign of geopathic stress or unhealthy underground energies. If you suspect this could be a possibility in your garden, consult a *feng shui* professional to advise on cures.

The positioning of trees in your garden is very important and large species should never be planted too close to the house. Not only will their *yin* influence be overpowering, but they will also create too much shade and their roots are likely to affect the foundations. For the same reasons, no tree should be allowed to grow taller than the house itself.

Trees to the front should generally be planted some distance away (depending on the species) if they are in line with the main entrance so that they do not block the passage of incoming *ch'i*. They can also be used as a protective barrier between the house and road but should not block out all sight of the street as this can lead to a sense of isolation or restriction.

Some *feng shui* practitioners believe creepers such as ivy on the walls of a house are inauspicious because brick or stonework needs to 'breathe' and if this process is blocked, it might lead to skin problems for the occupants. Others feel that the 'softening' effect of such plants is beneficial. As in most things, it is all a question of balance; grow climbers on your house if you wish but don't allow them to smother the facade and certainly keep them in check once they reach the eaves or gutters.

Where paths are narrow, avoid prickly plants such as roses, firethorn or *Berberis* in the adjacent beds; instead, use plants with rounded leaves which will not catch on passing flesh. If this is not possible, keep them trimmed so that they don't encroach on to the path. Plants with large spiky leaves such as yuccas should also be carefully placed so that the 'cutting' *ch'i* which emanates from their foliage will not cause problems. Keep them well away from paths and terraces so that there is plenty of surrounding space to negate their harmful energy.

Many plants can be related to *yin* and *yang* energy and also to the five elements. *Yang* plants grow upwards and have strong flower or foliage colour, whereas *yin* plants tend to be more floppy and grow downwards, with pale, softly coloured flowers and leaves. 'Water' plants tend to trail downwards or are clinging, while 'wood' plants appear solid and grow upwards, resembling the growth of trees. Plants with 'fire' energy have strong-coloured flowers and vertical form or pointed foliage, whereas 'earth' plants appear spreading and horizontal. 'Metal' energy is exhibited by plants with rounded leaves, flowers and forms. Use a balanced combination of plant types to create attractive groupings in terms of contrasting form, colour and texture. These will please the eye as well as ensuring harmonious energies in the garden.

Auspicious plants

Although plants in general symbolize healthy energy and good fortune, some are considered to be particularly auspicious and have their own individual meanings:

- peaches activate good health and lead to longevity
- bamboo also signifies good health and a long life
- pine trees and other conifers symbolize longevity: plant one for a baby boy to make him grow stronger
- plant a cherry tree for a baby girl to ensure a healthy and happy life
- chrysanthemums bring happiness into the home and are associated with a life of relaxation
- peonies are believed to be very auspicious for men, and strengthen their constitution

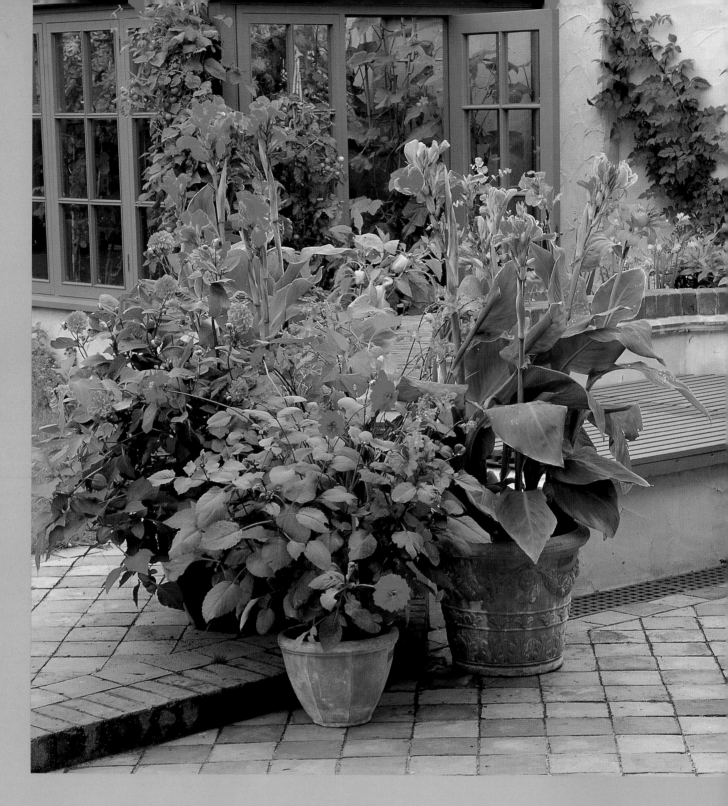

Red plants to activate *ch'i*

The potent red of these plants brings fire energy to the area, where it may be needed to counter an excess of metal (for instance where too much stone is causing disharmony), or to support earth where it might otherwise be weak or lacking. The *yang* nature of this colour will invigorate and lift the spirits. However, the temporary nature of these containers is probably a good thing: few people feel comfortable being exposed to red for too long.

Colours

Use colour in the garden in harmony with the concepts of *yin* and *yang* and the five elements. The colours linked with the elements can have a profound effect upon their surroundings. Many have quite different connotations to those in the West and their recommended use might therefore conflict with the advice given in the chapter on Colour therapy.

• Blue (water) denotes thoughtfulness, faith, caring and fidelity. Blue is *yin* and creates a very soothing atmosphere. Black also represents water and is an honourable colour although not often included in the garden; used in excess, it will reduce energy levels.

• Red (fire) is a most beneficial colour when used with care; it represents activity, life, strength, passion, happiness, good fortune and prosperity. Pink is a healthy colour which represents youth and romance; it also moderates anger. Almost as auspicious as red, purple is passionate and often linked to philosophy, dreaming, spiritual and artistic pursuits.

• Green (wood) is the colour of growth. It promotes healing and tranquillity and, when provided by plants, reflects peace and harmony which will ease a troubled mind. Green and red used in conjunction are very auspicious. Blue-greens tend towards *yin* and are relaxing yet still lively.

• White (metal) is the colour of old age and mourning in Chinese culture and is therefore not recommended for use in large areas on its own. All pale tints of colour have a particularly *yin* quality.

• Yellow (earth) signifies patience, tolerance, wisdom, fame and advancement. It brings inspiration and is warm and invigorating although not as hot as orange. Orange brightens up its surroundings and encourages togetherness; it also has healing powers.

Light

Lights bring 'fire' energy to any area and are especially beneficial when illuminating features being used as a 'cure', such as water, plants, or sculpture.

Mirrors

Mirrors can be put to good use to bring about a change in the energy of an area. They may be positioned to give the illusion of filling 'missing space', or used to activate the flow of *ch'i*, particularly when they reflect a 'cure'. A *pa kua* shaped (octagonal) mirror may be used to reflect away *sha ch'i* such as 'poison arrows'.

They must be kept clean at all times and should be placed flush against a wall. Always ensure that a pleasant view is reflected and avoid such items as rubbish bins or gloomy corners. Position mirrors carefully within the garden, since birds are often confused by what appears to be daylight and may fly into them.

Sound

In order to please all the senses, instruments such as wind chimes or bells have their place in the garden. Wind chimes are often used to moderate the flow of *ch'i* in areas where energy would otherwise have a tendency to rush straight through a space, for example along straight paths within a garden.

Always listen to them before buying so that you can choose a sound which appeals to you and will not annoy the neighbours.

Circular motion

Any feature which follows a circular movement is beneficial to the flow of energy. Mobiles, miniature windmills and fountains all fall into this category.

Heavy objects

In an area whose energy feels precarious or unbalanced, heavy boulders or sculptures can be used to stabilize the situation. Take care not to overdo this 'cure' as it could lead to stagnation.

Art

Many items of sculpture or statuary are suitable and can be used to 'activate' *ch'i* – symbolism has an important role to play. Always choose a piece with your intent in mind and select an image that appeals to you; in this regard it is a very personal matter.

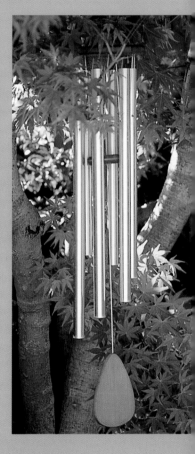

ABOVE Wind chimes are sometimes used to slow the flow of *ch'i* through an area, but are equally appropriate for simply bringing the added dimension of sound into the garden.

63

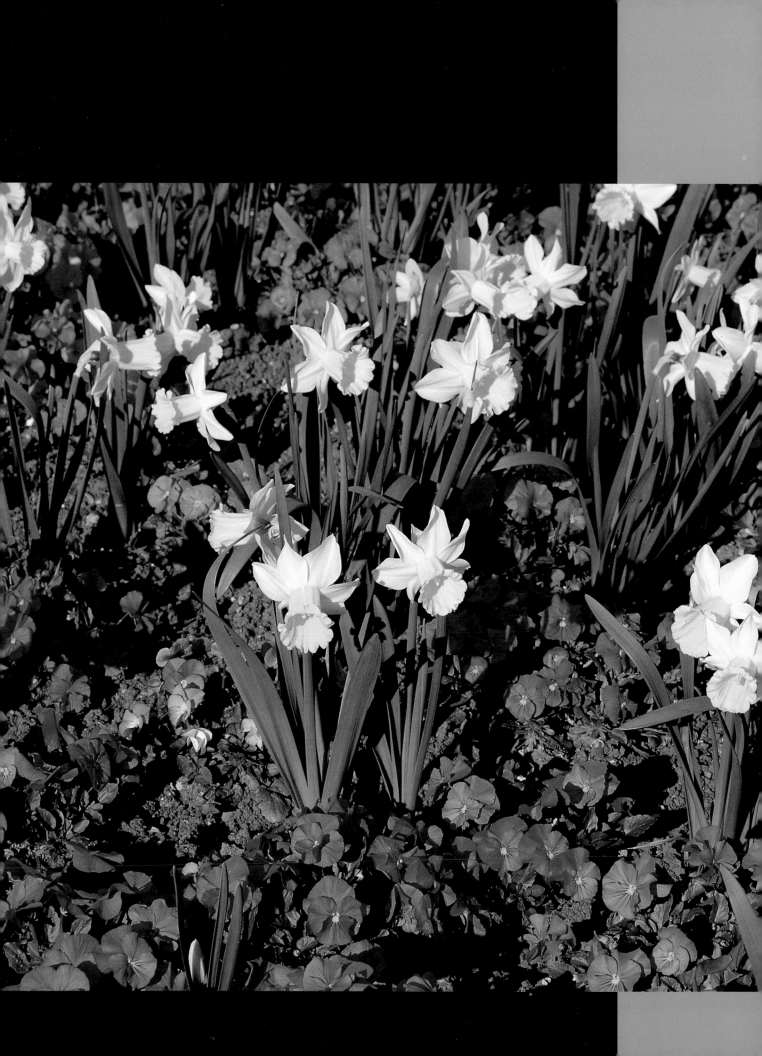

3

Colour therapy

Imagine that any mind ever thought a red geranium!
As if the redness of a red geranium
could be anything but a sensual experience
and as if sensual experience
could take place before there were any senses.
We know that even God
could not imagine the redness of a red geranium
nor the smell of mignonette
when geraniums were not, and mignonette neither.

D H LAWRENCE

Sight is the most immediate of all the physical senses. We do not have to do anything other than open our eyes to experience an ever-changing kaleidoscope of light and colour, which has a profound effect upon our well-being. While we make daily decisions about how to decorate our surroundings, we are often unaware of the impact they exert upon our physical and emotional states. Decades of research show that colour influences our thoughts, our actions, our health, and even our relationships with others. Indeed, many colour energies are so powerful that even the visually impaired can sense their vibrations and identify a colour simply by 'feeling' the density of the air that surrounds it.

Colour therapy is an ancient approach to healing that has been used since the earliest of times. As with other holistic treatments, it aims to restore harmony and stimulate the patient's inner resources to aid the recovery of health, the fundamental belief being that illness develops from imbalances of energies at emotional, spiritual or physical levels.

Treatment with colour was probably first practised by the ancient Egyptians, who shone sunlight through coloured gems on to those who sought healing. The practice of healing through colour is also known to have been adopted in ancient Greece, India, Tibet and China, by the Mayans of Central America and the Native North Americans. (Even today, practitioners of Chinese medicine believe that colours have a profound effect upon health and that illness can be diagnosed

LEFT As direct opposites on the colour wheel, violet and yellow create a powerful complementary contrast. In this instance, winter-flowering pansies and daffodils provide a splash of early colour in the garden; if space is limited, both would be equally well suited to a windowbox.

through the colour of certain parts of the body, including the tongue.)

However, as with herbalism, aromatherapy and many other ancient healing arts, colour therapy all but disappeared in the West. It was not until the eighteenth century that scientists and artists began to revive interest in the properties of light and colour. Study has continued throughout the nineteenth and twentieth centuries, and the philosopher and educationalist Rudolf Steiner (1861–1925) developed some theories of colour therapy that are widely accepted today. Although the effect of colour in interior design is now well documented, little advice is available regarding our outdoor environment. This chapter aims to take some of these healing techniques into the garden.

Colour for healing

While some of the theory behind colour therapy remains scientifically unproven, studies have demonstrated that colours can profoundly affect mood and often have a measurable effect on the emotional and physical behaviour of human beings. The range of chronic and acute health issues treated by therapists is extensive and improvement is claimed in such conditions as migraine, asthma, eczema, depression, lethargy, the common cold, high and low blood pressure, arthritis, rheumatism and many mental and emotional problems. Colour treatment has been found to be especially useful in stress-related disorders such as eczema and mild depression. It is particularly valuable when used to support other therapies and is often practised alongside conventional medicine.

Our psychological response plays a vital role in colour healing, many colours having powerful emotional and spiritual undertones as well as physical implications. Throughout our lives we attach feelings, memories and meanings to our experience of colour and these associations build up our personal colour preferences. Many of us have strong leanings towards certain colours, and the origins of favourite and disliked colours are considered very important in healing; therapists often

find we avoid a much needed colour simply because of its unpleasant past associations. Although personal taste is significant, it does appear that most people prefer colours in the so-called 'universal order' of blue, red, green, violet, yellow, orange. However, underlying preferences can also be affected by the influences of fashion.

Colour therapists initially analyse a patient through a variety of techniques to diagnose whether he or she is 'off-colour'. Illness is seen as a lack of one or more colours within the body, where each colour has specific characteristics and effects. Although invisible to most people, every natural being is surrounded by an energy field which can be seen as an enveloping aura. The aura is a continually moving and pulsing entity, holding life energy and reflecting physical and mental state. In a healthy person, all the colours of the spectrum are visible, from red nearest the body through to the outer band of magenta. This same life force also shines through the chakras – energy centres within the body which are closely linked to the function of internal organs and systems.

Mental, physical and emotional trauma is reflected by imbalances within the aura, which colour therapists seek to harmonize by the application of missing colour(s). In this way, healing is encouraged before subtle instabilities manifest as more serious illness. Every colour contains energy of a certain vibration and each organ in the body is linked with a corresponding colour; controlled exposure to an appropriate colour can therefore correct or enhance the body's energy flow. Extremes of emotion, which we all acknowledge when we use phrases like 'green with envy', are often the outward display of imbalances or blockages in the flow of colour energies into and out of the body.

Different colours affect the amount and type of light that falls on us. Colour, in the form of light energy, enters not only through the eyes, but also the skin, which we do not consciously register. It permeates through the aura, triggering chemical and hormonal changes within the body which affect health and well-being. Exposure to certain colours can therefore adjust our intake of light energy, in order to balance the body. Even the colour blind or visually impaired can be healed with colour as the treatment does not have to be seen.

Imbalances are corrected through a variety of techniques, exposure to the colour or colours lasting approximately twenty minutes. Patients may be treated with special lamps, crystals, coloured silks, colourful food or liquids, or through the use of coloured oils for massage. Any treatment is enhanced by total relaxation. Taking the garden as our healing environment, we shall examine suitable techniques to adopt outdoors.

Colour and light

Sir Isaac Newton (1643–1727) was the first to discover that light could be broken up into the component colours of the spectrum, from red to violet, when shone through a triangular prism. He identified an extra colour, indigo, in order to classify seven colours (since this was considered a 'mystical' number) and was also the first to devise a colour wheel that included all the colours of the spectrum in the correct sequence.

In the twentieth century, much of the mysticism has been stripped away from the subject as Einstein demonstrated that light behaved in a much more complex way than was previously thought.

Visible light was found to be part of a wider spectrum of electromagnetic energy, which includes radiowaves, X-rays, microwaves and gamma radiation. In the same way that a radio receives energy waves of a certain frequency and converts them into sound, the eye receives light waves between 400 million million cycles per second (violet) and 800 million million cycles per second (red), which the brain converts to colour. The narrow band of energy detected by the human eye lies in the middle of the electromagnetic spectrum.

Such energy is believed to travel in waves, each minute shift in wavelength being sensed by the eye and interpreted as a different colour. The energy of full spectrum white light contains all the wavelengths of colour. Too much or too little light can upset general health, as can the type of light. For example,

SAD (Seasonal Affective Disorder) is linked with the widespread use of artificial lighting throughout winter; such light has none of the variety of natural light and deprives us of certain colour energies.

How we see colour

The eye works like a camera, its lens focusing the light rays and the iris controlling the amount of light that falls on the retina at the back of the eye. The retina contains light receptors of two types – cones and rods. Cones are active in daylight and convey colour sensation; they can be subdivided into three types, each containing a pigment sensitive only to red, blue or green. Rods are sensitive only to intensity of light and are therefore responsible for night vision. Rod and cone cells convert the light energy received by the eye into electrical impulses which travel down some one million nerve fibres leading from the retina to the optic nerve. The optic nerve then conveys messages to the visual cortex in the brain for interpretation in terms of sight – colour, relative lightness and form.

Some of these nervous impulses trigger the hypothalamus, a biological control centre which regulates sleep, hunger, thirst, temperature and other involuntary functions. The hypothalamus also influences the pituitary and pineal glands in the brain, which control other functions of the body by producing hormones that stimulate such diverse areas as the adrenal glands and reproductive organs. Thus the metabolism of the entire body is affected.

The various wavelengths of light energy are reflected back to the retina from the objects they strike and the information is interpreted by the brain into various hues. A pure white surface reflects almost all light rays, which then combine on the retina to appear white. Pure red pigment absorbs orange, yellow, green, blue and violet rays, so that only the reflected red rays reach the eye and are consequently seen as red. Colour perception is affected both by the quality of light and the texture of the object.

We see the colour of an object first and after registering the hue, the eye then decodes its other

RIGHT Here, again, is a good example of complementary contrast, this time in blue and orange. Each colour makes the other, its opposite, appear even more intense than it would if set against any other colour in the spectrum. In colour therapy, it is important that you include the complementary contrast of the colour you wish to use for healing in your planting scheme to ensure you receive a balanced treatment and do not 'overdose' on your selected colour.

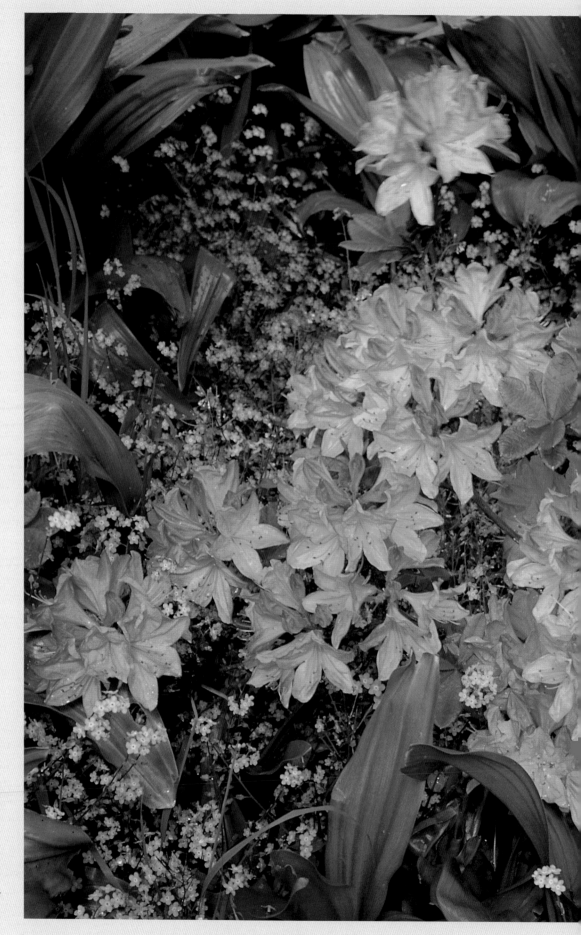

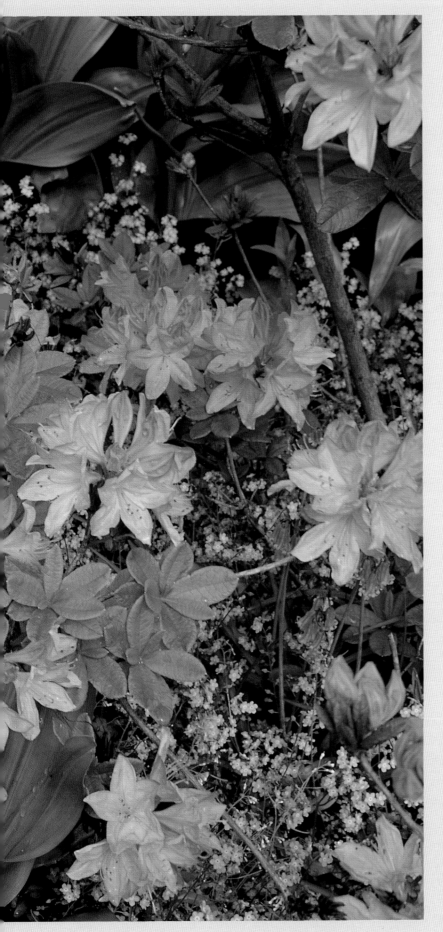

properties, for instance light and shade, tone and saturation. Yellow or yellow-green light naturally focuses directly on to the retina and is therefore the colour we perceive most easily. Red light waves are longer and focus at a point behind the retina, causing the lens to become convex in order to focus. This gives the sensation of pulling the colour nearer and so red, when seen with other colours, seems to advance in front of them. Shorter blue light tends to focus in front of the retina so the lens has to turn concave and this gives the illusion of pushing the colour back. Therefore blue seems to recede in comparison with other colours.

While we may understand how the brain deciphers the colour 'messages' received from the eye, there are unexplained reactions which seem to take place within the mind. The concept of 'after image' or 'successive contrast' is one such example. If we stare at a primary colour for a minute and then look at a white area, we will see a 'ghost' image in the complementary colour. Another phenomenon is that of 'simultaneous contrast', where two colours placed side by side will be tinged with the haze of their neighbour's complementary colour. For instance, if blue and yellow are placed side by side the blue will be tinged with violet and an orange tint will deepen the yellow. This helps to explain why complementary colours have such a powerful effect when used together – each colour becomes the antithesis of the other (see next page).

The perception of colour may therefore be considered a mental and psychological phenomenon as well as a physical one. It involves a highly complex and largely subjective interaction between the eye and the brain. While we may physically focus the eye, the brain then takes over and uses its own experience to decipher what it actually sees, and then what to call it. In this way, the effects of colour are often confused by mood, memory and other psychological factors whereby the brain will assume what the eye is seeing. None of us sees colour in quite the same way, or to the same intensity. We may think of colour simply in physical terms but it is active at all levels: mental, emotional and spiritual.

The theory of colour

Throughout the nineteenth and twentieth centuries, there has been a great deal of research into the dynamics of colour. Most scientists and artists working with colour agree that there are six basic hues: three primary (red, yellow and blue) and three secondary (green, orange and violet). The three primary hues are thus named because they cannot be created by mixing other pigments. Two primary colours will combine to create a secondary colour and tertiary colours are formed by mixing a primary with a secondary colour to create another six colours. For instance, yellow and green combine to produce yellow-green, blue and violet create blue-violet. We will stop here for simplicity's sake, but this categorization continues *ad infinitum*, since people with normal eyesight are able to differentiate up to ten million different hues and, with practice, most can sharpen the eye even further.

Colour practitioners often work with nine colours: red, orange, yellow, green, blue, indigo, violet, magenta and turquoise. To keep things simple and make the best use of the colour available in the garden, we shall study only the six primary and secondary colours: red, orange, yellow, green, blue and violet.

COLOUR WHEEL For ease of use, the colour spectrum is normally portrayed as a wheel. This wheel is one of the basic tools used in the analysis of colour.

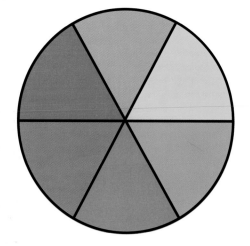

Mixing colours

When colours are placed together, the relationship between them is as important as the colours themselves; when seen in combination they will always be modified in some way. The eye has a tendency to exaggerate the differences between adjacent colours, while colours tend to retain their truest appearance beside white (or grey); this is worth bearing in mind when finding a spot for treatment in the garden. It may be advisable to paint the surrounding walls or fences white so that the planting is not adversely affected by adjacent brickwork or wood stains.

The most intense contrasts are created by pairing the three primary and three secondary colours thus: red/green, yellow/violet and blue/orange. The paired colours together create a balanced whole. This concept is closely linked to the theory of *yin* and *yang* – that everything in the universe has an equal and opposite and each contains within it the potential for the other.

When working with complementary pairs, some hues appear more dominant than others and care needs to be taken to compose a harmonious balance. A mix of approximately 70% healing colour to 30% complementary colour is generally recommended for treatments. However, yellow and orange have a tendency to overpower their partners, violet and blue, and the ratio may need to be adjusted to achieve a feeling of balance. Red and green are more tonally similar and have an equal influence.

In addition, some colours appear to advance while others retreat, an effect created by the focusing of the retina (see previous page). The warm tones of red and orange will tend to advance in front of cooler tones such as blue, green or violet and this can play havoc with the desired result. For this reason, relative quantities of orange and red, when used as contrasts to blue and green, may need to be reduced to prevent them overpowering the healing colour. Much of the above will depend upon individual circumstances and it may be a matter of trial and error to find an acceptable equilibrium.

RIGHT The concept of complementary pairs of colours can sometimes be illustrated by a single plant. Here, ruby chard displays an incredible combination of red and green which you might not normally expect to find in nature.

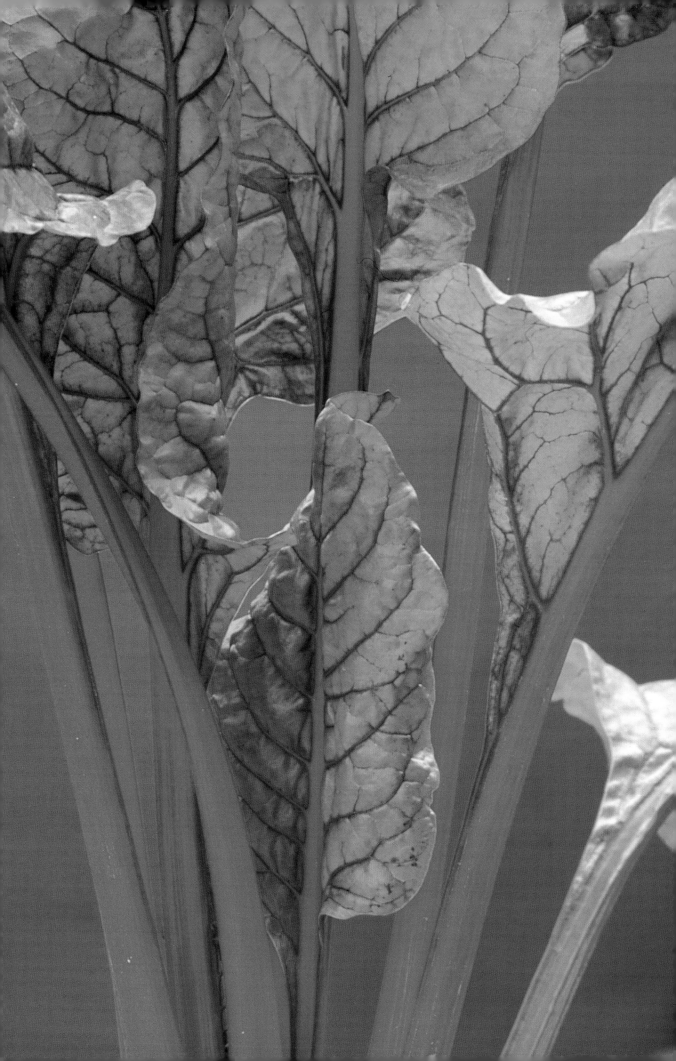

Colour in the garden

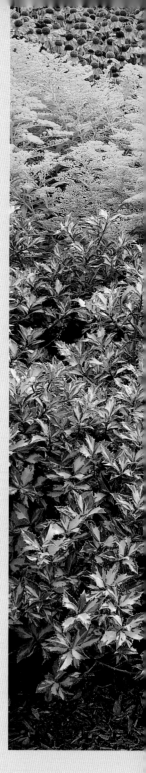

The availability of colour for our gardens has never been wider than it is today. Plant breeders continue to produce flowers and foliage in almost every imaginable hue and we can now buy materials, paints and accessories in every colour of the spectrum. Yet many gardens are still dominated by grey or beige concrete, insipid pastel flowers and dull green foliage. It often seems that we are afraid to use bold colour, perhaps believing that soft earthy tones are most appropriate in the garden. I believe that we are wasting wonderful opportunities to use the healing power of colour in our gardens.

Each colour has many meanings and abilities and can heal a wide variety of conditions. There is no 'best' colour for healing and the choice should be an entirely personal one. Therapists believe that we are often instinctively drawn towards the colour that we most need and so perhaps we simply need to learn to trust our inner feelings.

A healthy aura (the invisible energy field that surrounds every living being) contains a balance of colours and for this reason, both complementary colours must always be used in a treatment or the condition could actually be worsened. Plantings for colour healing within the garden will therefore include closely related tones of the chosen hue and a smaller amount (about one third) of the complementary colour, which should be introduced in blocks throughout the area.

The colour impact will rely more upon overall effect than the individual shade of each flower. The relationship between the plants themselves and that with their wider surroundings need to be considered. There may be some garden situations where common sense dictates that certain colours might be overwhelming or unsuitable, but the effects of a particularly bright hue can always be mitigated through careful positioning and possibly screening.

It should also be remembered that the green foliage in larger planting beds will inevitably predominate. The choice of suitable plants will therefore be dictated both by the strength of flower or foliage colour and by the quantity of flowers produced.

Our perception of colour within the garden shifts constantly as the sun moves across the sky and we enjoy the dynamics of passing time. As any artist knows, the most constant light is north-facing but unfortunately, choosing such a position would restrict the range of plants that could be grown. On the other hand, strong sunlight can add a yellow tinge to everything and make it difficult to focus on particularly bright colours. It is therefore advisable to place your seating area and planting in light shade in order to gain maximum benefit from the widest possible choice of plants. At dusk, violets, reds and blues become more sober and paler shades of yellow come into their own.

Gardeners also need to take account of the variations in flower colour that occur naturally in different soil conditions. A well-known example is hydrangeas, where the pH value of the soil is reflected in the flower colour, but many other plants are similarly, albeit more subtly, affected.

The siting of an area for colour healing will depend to a certain extent upon the basic structure of the garden. A large garden might permit the construction of a number of distinct areas, each with its own colour, and it may make sense to retain a permanent framework of foliage plants and alter the flowering plants as required. A small town garden or terrace can fulfil your requirements equally well and even a window box can serve a useful purpose. In a smaller garden, you can change your chosen colour on an annual basis if desired, simply by replanting a group of containers and repainting accessories where necessary. If a neutral background of white or a

ABOVE This border contains a number of plants selected for their yellow flowers and foliage, among them golden rod (*Solidago*), holly (*Ilex*) and sneezewort (*Helenium*). The purple verbena flowers in the foreground provide the necessary contrast colour in about the right quantity.

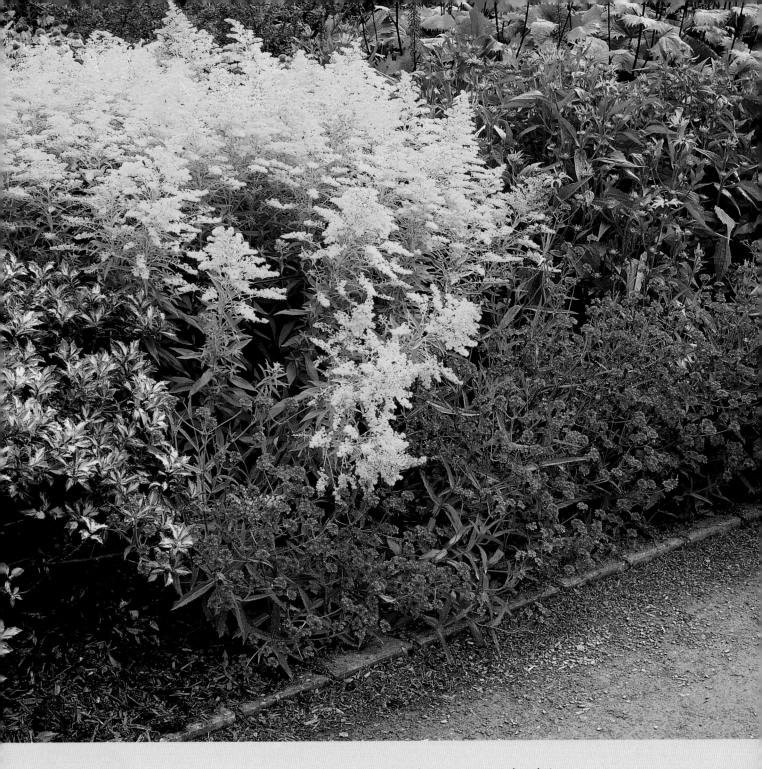

greyish tone is used, it is possible to change the hue of the planting from season to season, perhaps to suit your changing health needs. Temporary displays of annuals may be used to supplement or extend the permanent planting.

The impact of colour will depend not only upon the relative size of the area but also the distance from which it is seen. It is preferable to sit as close to the planting as possible to gain the full benefit. If there is room in the garden, you might be able to sit within the chosen area, totally immersed in colour. In a smaller garden, it might simply be a matter of

grouping containers close to a seat so that their impact is more tangible.

Monochrome planting schemes – attractive in themselves but without the potential for healing – can teach us many lessons about the use of a limited colour palette. They rely upon factors such as form, shape and texture to prevent the scene from becoming a boring mass. Aim to establish a balanced composition, using solid plants for background and structure, with horizontal and vertical contrasts, juxtapositions of rounded and spiky shapes, and some more ethereal foliage and flowers.

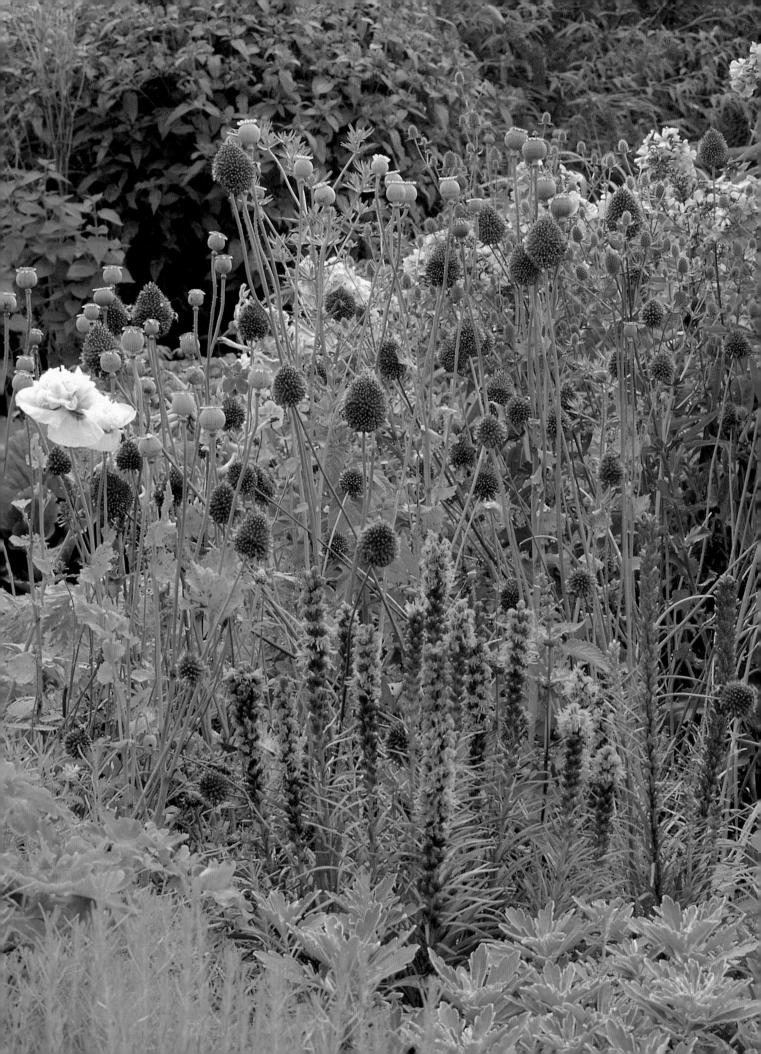

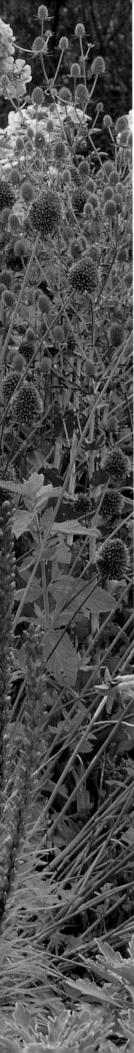

LEFT Purple can be a difficult colour to use en masse as certain hues have a tendency toward dullness. Such a border can be enlivened by using a range of tones, from pinks to blues, and including a variety of textures. Here, the drumstick flowers of *Allium sphaerocephalon* stand out against the spikes of *Liatris spicata,* while the mass of purple-tinted flowers of sea holly (*Eryngium*) and *Phlox paniculata* 'Franz Schubert' create a harmonious background. For colour healing, a splash of yellow would complete the picture – very little would be required as yellow has a tendency to dominate its surroundings.

Although the colour(s) chosen will depend largely upon personal health requirements, the size and style of the garden, colours of house materials and type of neighbourhood do need to be borne in mind. The usual rules of garden design apply, and aspect, scale and privacy must be considered. To ensure compatibility, a little knowledge of the natural ecology of the plants will prove useful in order to satisfy their cultural needs.

Certain colours act as focal points, dominating or attracting attention; others – specifically those with bluish tones – will increase the sense of space by fading into the background. The apparent size of the garden can thus be manipulated, increasing space in a small garden or creating a more cosy atmosphere in a larger one. The brighter hues of red, orange and yellow need particularly careful placement so as not to jar in a rural landscape; it is normally advisable to keep such colours closer to the house. Once the location and colour of the area has been set, why stop with the garden? It often makes sense to link the colours of the garden with your interior decor.

When embarking on the selection of plants, it is important to choose those you like, not simply the ones that fulfil your basic requirements. As you decide on plants for your desired colour effects, consider also their appearance during the seasons outside their main period of interest. What may initially appear to be a bewilderingly large range of suitable plants can be rapidly whittled down.

It will inevitably be harder to provide for certain colours throughout the year than others. In temperate climates we enjoy distinct seasonal colour associations. We expect spring colours to be refreshing shades of yellow, blue and lime green and know that later summer colours will become richer and stronger, giving way to fiery autumn tones and finally the browns and greys of winter. It may well be that an orange garden will be most powerful during autumn, while violet will be hard to find during winter. Although such limitations may be frustrating at times, there will always be possibilities, especially if you look beyond flowers to foliage, fruit, berries, bark and stems.

Don't overlook the value of materials and accessories in the colour garden. Furniture and other decorative items can be relied upon to add colour when plants are lacking. Paving in red brick, golden gravel, yellow stone or blue slate can harmonize or contrast with the chosen hue. Glazed pots are available in every imaginable colour and can be planted to produce stunning arrangements. All materials should, if possible, be of natural origin: clay pavers, natural stone and terracotta pots are all preferable to concrete.

Another valuable asset is a canvas parasol or awning. This can be dyed in almost any colour and the light cast through it will bathe you in a healing glow, supplementing the colour provided by other garden elements.

Red for vitality

Red is the colour of love and fertility and is a great energizer. It keeps you alert, helps you cope with the demands of life, removes negativity and provides courage. Representing strength of will, with a drive that pushes you on to greater things, its energy is a useful pick-me-up if you are depressed or tired and it can rescue you from the brink of hopelessness. Some, however, may find it too stimulating when under pressure and it can aggravate stress, causing anger to surface.

Along with blue, red is the colour most often chosen in colour preference tests. However, a dislike of red is fairly common and this is often characteristic of someone who has been frustrated or defeated.

Many people find pink more comfortable than a bright red; this may demonstrate a lack of courage. Pink is also chosen by those seeking affection and has the ability to engender unconditional love. It is also helpful to those suffering from grief, since it protects and brings peace of mind.

Exposure to red causes measurable reactions in the body. Blood pressure, temperature and energy levels are raised, circulation improves and breathing, pulse rate and brainwave action quickens. These are only temporary effects and quickly die down when the colour is withdrawn. Red strengthens the blood and therefore helps treat anaemia. It is also a detoxifier, removing debris from both the psyche and the body, and will help to fight off infection. Red raises comfort levels, making cold areas feel a few degrees warmer than they actually are, so it is a very useful colour for those who catch colds easily or who need warmth. It is a real support when you feel sluggish or apathetic, providing physical and mental energy. An arousing colour, it is not suitable for the treatment of anxiety or emotional disturbance.

Red is the colour of the base chakra, the energy centre within the body that is associated with the lower trunk and reproductive organs. For this reason, it is believed to be helpful in the treatment of genital problems and issues of sexuality or infertility. It can also ease stiff limbs, particularly the legs.

Red in the garden

The boldest and most eye-catching colour in the garden, red commands attention and provides vibrancy, making areas seem smaller than they actually are because of its 'advancing' nature. No matter what the shade of red, the essential energy is never lost; it is most often found in late summer and autumn, when it seems to take over almost every plant. Due to its ability to increase appetite, red is a good colour to use around dining areas and would also be suitable for other spaces where activity is to be encouraged.

Materials which might be used to augment the planting include glazed pots, red sandstone gravels and red clay bricks, tiles or pavers.

Red plants Complementary colour: green

In spring and summer, temporary bursts of red may be provided by pansies, nasturtium, pelargoniums, salvias, verbena or busy lizzies. The list of flowering plants is supplemented by those whose leaves, bark, berries and bare stems bring splashes of red into the garden in autumn and winter.

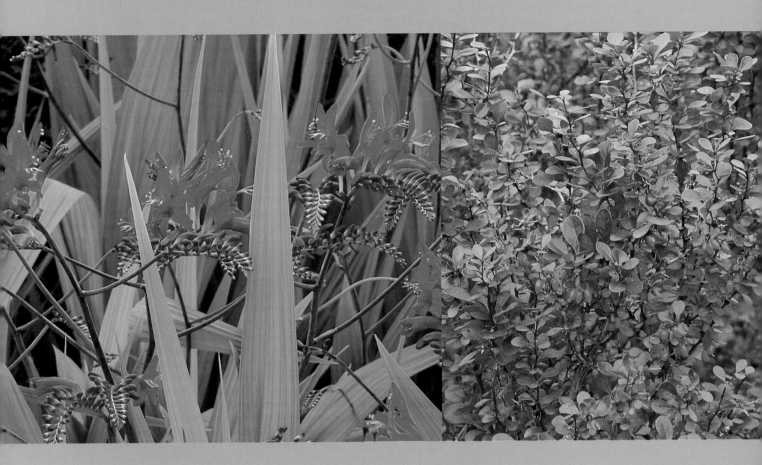

LEFT The stunning red flowers of *Crocosmia* 'Lucifer' provide valuable late summer colour.

RIGHT Although the foliage of *Berberis thunbergii* 'Red Pillar' is red throughout the year, in autumn it really glows as the leaves turn a vivid scarlet.

Spring

Chaenomeles x superba 'Crimson and Gold' (JAPANESE QUINCE)
Cytisus 'Burkwoodii' (BROOM)
Erysimum cheiri 'Blood Red' (WALLFLOWER)
Magnolia liliiflora 'Nigra' (MAGNOLIA)
Malus x purpurea 'Lemoinei' (CRAB APPLE)
Photinia x fraseri 'Red Robin' (foliage)
Rhododendron 'Elizabeth'
Ribes speciosum (FLOWERING CURRANT)
Syringa vulgaris 'Souvenir de Louis Spaeth' (LILAC)
Tulipa 'Balalaika' (TULIP)

Summer

Clematis 'Niobe'
Cosmos atrosanguineus (CHOCOLATE PLANT)
Dianthus ' Queen of Hearts' (PINK)
Fuchsia 'Mrs Popple'
Hemerocallis 'Stafford' (DAY LILY)
Paeonia officinalis (PEONY)
Papaver orientale 'Goliath' (ORIENTAL POPPY)
Penstemon 'Garnet'
Primula japonica 'Miller's Crimson'
Rosa 'Parkdirektor Riggers' (ROSE)

Autumn

Berberis thunbergii atropurpurea (BARBERRY – foliage, berries)
Buddleja davidii 'Royal Red' (BUTTERFLY BUSH)
Clematis 'Madame Julia Correvon'
Cotinus coggygria 'Royal Purple' (SMOKE BUSH)
Crocosmia 'Lucifer' (MONTBRETIA)
Euonymus alatus (WINGED SPINDLE)
Hydrangea quercifolia (OAK-LEAVED HYDRANGEA)
Parthenocissus tricuspidata 'Veitchii' (BOSTON IVY)
Viburnum opulus (GUELDER ROSE – foliage, berries)
Vitis coignetiae (GRAPE VINE)

Winter

Bergenia 'Margery Fish' (ELEPHANTS' EARS)
Camellia japonica 'Adolphe Audusson'
Cornus alba 'Sibirica' (DOGWOOD – stems)
Erica carnea 'Eileen Porter' (WINTER HEATH)
Ilex aquifolium 'J C Van Tol' (HOLLY– berries)
Phormium 'Dazzler' (NEW ZEALAND FLAX – foliage)
Prunus serrula (CHERRY – bark)
Pyracantha 'Mohave' (FIRETHORN – berries)
Salix alba 'Chermesina' (WILLOW – bark)
Skimmia japonica (berries)

Orange for optimism

Orange is primarily the colour of joy; exposure to it promotes a feeling of well-being by providing a release from the everyday worries of life. Warm and welcoming, optimistic and sociable, it is bursting with earthly energy and will act as a stimulant to those in its presence, albeit with a gentler effect than that of red. Orange provokes change, creates opportunity and is the colour of activity, enthusiasm and freedom. It deals with dormant conditions by bringing them into the open so that they can be sorted out and properly laid to rest. It is a good colour for putting your life back together again when grieving, divorced or in shock and is often used for mental breakdowns or suicidal feelings. If used appropriately, its healing properties may be harnessed to lift the spirits, combat depression and fight unknown fears.

Preferred by the quick-witted and talkative, orange is also a colour often chosen in tests by those suffering from mental or physical exhaustion, perhaps signifying a subconscious desire for a less stressful life. Orange is a popular colour with children and is used in classrooms for younger children in Steiner schools, where it is believed to encourage resourcefulness and independence, while improving social behaviour by lessening hostility and irritability.

Orange is the colour of the sacral chakra, the energy centre within the body that is associated with the adrenal glands, the lower intestines, the abdomen, kidneys and bladder. Orange improves intestinal disorders and bowel disturbance and also helps to increase the appetite, since it is associated with the assimilation of food. It is thought to be a good aid to the menopause (both male and female) as it balances the hormones. Orange may also be used in the treatment of the following: arthritis, asthma, bronchitis, catarrh, fibroids, gallstones, hip problems, impotence, infertility, knee problems, muscle cramps or spasms, underactive thyroid.

Orange in the garden

Although not as potent as red, orange nevertheless requires careful treatment in the garden. It is a powerful and strident colour, particularly in a rural environment where it can often appear out of place. In small gardens it will tend to have a foreshortening effect and can be overpowering if not handled with restraint. The richest hues may be found in the flowers, ripe fruit and autumn leaves of late summer and autumn, but it is a colour found widely in nature.

In our homes, orange is appropriate for a dining area or space used for entertainment, relating as it does to enjoyment and movement. In the garden we could consider using it for a barbecue area or around a terrace used for eating. Orange may also be used to provide a lift at the start of the day and is an excellent choice for an area in which to enjoy a cup of tea in the morning sun. Furniture and accessories can provide much of the colour, with container-grown plants to introduce seasonal highlights.

Many materials commonly included in the garden can supplement the colour provided by plants; these might take the form of terracotta pots and ornaments, rusting metals, warm golden gravels and the earthy tones of clay brick.

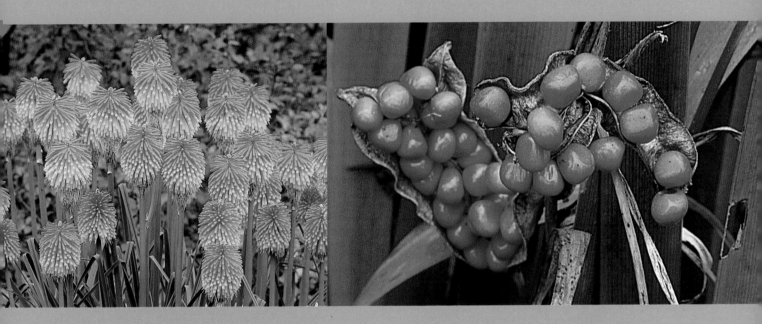

Orange plants Complementary colour: blue

To enhance the effect throughout the year, gaps in permanent garden plantings may be filled by pansies, ranunculus, gazania, nasturtium, marigolds, mimulus or zinnia. After the flowers of spring and summer and the berries of autumn, the bark of certain trees remains orange throughout the winter.

LEFT The flowers of *Kniphofia rooperi* (red hot poker) appear throughout late summer and autumn above clumps of sword-like foliage.

RIGHT Of particular value in the depths of winter are the orange berries of stinking iris (*Iris foetidissima*), which are revealed as the pods burst open.

Spring

Berberis darwinii (BARBERRY)

Chaenomeles japonica (FLOWERING QUINCE)

Crocus 'Golden Bunch'

Euphorbia griffithii 'Fireglow' (SPURGE)

Fritillaria imperialis 'Orange Brilliant' (FRITILLARY)

Narcissus 'Delibes' (DAFFODIL)

Papaver orientale 'Harvest Moon' (ORIENTAL POPPY)

Primula bulleyana (CANDELABRA PRIMULA)

Rhododendron 'Gibraltar' (AZALEA)

Tulipa 'Orange Emperor' (TULIP)

Summer

Alstroemeria aurea (PERUVIAN LILY)

Campsis radicans (TRUMPET VINE)

Eschscholzia californica (CALIFORNIAN POPPY)

Geum 'Borisii'

Hemerocallis fulva 'Florepleno' (DAY LILY)

Kniphofia rooperi (RED HOT POKER)

Lilium 'Enchantment' (LILY)

Lonicera sempervirens (HONEYSUCKLE)

Potentilla fruticosa 'Tangerine'

Rosa foetida 'Bicolor' (ROSE)

Autumn

Acer capillipes (SNAKE BARK MAPLE)

Amelanchier lamarckii (SNOWY MESPILUS – foliage)

Cotinus coggygria (SMOKE BUSH – foliage)

Hippophae rhamnoides (SEA BUCKTHORN – berries)

Hypericum x inodorum 'Elstead' (ST JOHN'S WORT – berries)

Malus 'John Downie' (CRAB APPLE – fruit)

Rhus typhina (STAG'S HORN SUMACH – foliage)

Rosa rugosa (ROSE – fruit)

Taxodium distichum (SWAMP CYPRESS)

Viburnum opulus 'Xanthocarpum' (GUELDER ROSE – foliage, berries)

Winter

Acer griseum (PAPERBARK MAPLE)

Betula albosinensis var. *septentrionalis* (BIRCH – bark)

Cotoneaster x suecicus 'Coral Beauty' (berries)

Cryptomeria japonica 'Elegans' (JAPANESE CEDAR – foliage)

Erica carnea 'Ruby Glow' (WINTER HEATH)

Hamamelis x intermedia 'Jelena' (WITCH HAZEL)

Ilex aquifolium 'Amber' (HOLLY – berries)

Iris foetidissima (STINKING IRIS – berries)

Prunus serrula (CHERRY – bark)

Pyracantha 'Orange Glow' (FIRETHORN – berries)

Yellow for contentment

Yellow, the brightest colour in the spectrum, represents the power of the sun. A great aid to concentration and study, yellow energy provides intellectual and inspirational stimulation, encourages agility of mind, aids precision of thought and absorption of facts and helps to sort out difficulties. However, some colour therapists believe an excess of yellow may be too stressful a stimulant and that it should be used with caution. Yellow is also a useful colour for the shy or the lonely as it brings feelings of optimism and self-worth and lifts depression. It encourages detachment and allows you to stand back from a situation and think your own way through it.

Often selected by intelligent people who like innovation, yellow is also liked by the mentally handicapped. Those who dislike yellow often feel isolated or have suffered disappointment.

Its energy is a powerful eliminator, purging waste from the body and toning and cleansing the entire system. This is not only of physical benefit but also applies to emotional baggage, since holistic medicine believes that illness often stems from the stress of holding on to unresolved situations and not letting go of old problems.

The solar plexus is governed by yellow and also the liver, pancreas, gall bladder, spleen and middle stomach; therefore yellow is of general benefit to the digestive system. Used for weight control, it helps to maintain a correct balance of liquids in the body, alleviating water retention. It also works on the skin and can benefit the treatment of eczema and psoriasis. Yellow seems to prevent calcium accumulating in the joints of older people, which eases arthritis and rheumatism. It provides a boost to the nervous system, keeping the nerves strong and generating muscle energy.

The following may also respond to yellow energy: allergies, cellulite, high blood cholesterol levels, poor circulation, constipation, cystitis, depression, diabetes, ear problems and tinnitus, hair loss, myalgic encephalomyelitis (ME), and even leukaemia and stroke (the latter should be undertaken in conjunction with conventional treatment).

Yellow in the garden

Yellow is a powerful colour and will attract and dominate, drawing the eye toward it. It also increases the feeling of space, which means areas may be difficult to define and much of the detail can be lost. If used to excess, plants with yellow or golden variegated foliage can merge into an unsightly jumble; it is therefore important to vary texture and form, including strong vertical and horizontal accents where appropriate. Since the golden foliage of many plants will scorch in full sunshine, such an area will generally require light shade; this also has the effect of making the plants appear more luminous.

Yellow will bring a sense of well-being to the garden even on a dull day. It evokes the spirit of spring and calls to mind the vibrant hues of daffodils and forsythia and the pale yellow-green shoots of young foliage. Many grey or 'silver'-leaved plants have yellow flowers.

Materials to use in the yellow garden include reconstituted stone containers and ornaments, golden sandstone gravels and buff paving.

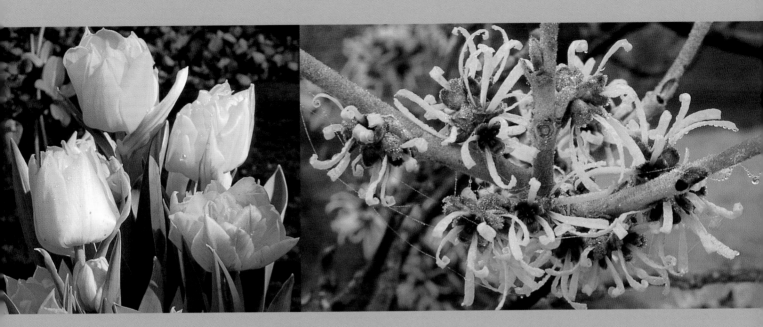

Yellow plants Complementary colour: violet

Annuals which will enhance the effect throughout the year include pansies, primroses, wallflowers, ranunculus, snapdragons, marigolds, marguerites, nasturtium. After spring and summer flowers, many plants have yellow berries and bark for autumn and winter colour.

LEFT Spring is heralded by the arrival of flowering bulbs such as this double yellow tulip (*Tulipa* 'Monte Carlo').

RIGHT Your spirits cannot fail to be lifted in mid-winter by the appearance of the fragrant, spidery flowers of witch hazel (*Hamamelis mollis*).

Spring

Caltha palustris 'Plena' (MARSH MARIGOLD)
Crocus chrysanthus 'E A Bowles'
Euphorbia polychroma (SPURGE)
Forsythia x intermedia 'Lynwood'
Hakonechloa macra 'Aureola' (foliage)
Narcissus 'Golden Rapture' (DAFFODIL)
Paeonia lutea var. *ludlowii* (TREE PEONY)
Prunus 'Ukon' (FLOWERING CHERRY)
Rhododendron luteum (AZALEA)
Rosa banksiae 'Lutea' (BANKSIAN ROSE)

Summer

Achillea 'Moonshine' (YARROW)
Cytisus x praecox (BROOM)
Hemerocallis 'Towhead' (DAY LILY)
Humulus lupulus 'Aureus' (GOLDEN HOP – foliage)
Lonicera japonica 'Halliana' (HONEYSUCKLE)
Oenothera biennis (EVENING PRIMROSE)
Phlomis fruticosa (JERUSALEM SAGE)
Pleioblastus auricomus (BAMBOO – foliage)
Potentilla fruticosa 'Elizabeth'
Rosa 'Golden Wings' (ROSE)

Autumn

Clematis tangutica
Cotoneaster salicifolius 'Exburyensis' (berries)
Cupressus macrocarpa 'Goldcrest' (CYPRESS – foliage)
Ginkgo biloba (MAIDENHAIR TREE – foliage)
Helenium 'Butterpat' (SNEEZEWORT)
Hypericum 'Hidcote' (ST JOHN'S WORT)
Lilium auratum (JAPANESE GOLDEN-RAYED LILY)
Pyracantha 'Soleil d'Or' (FIRETHORN – berries)
Rudbeckia fulgida 'Goldsturm' (CONEFLOWER)
Sorbus 'Joseph Rock' (MOUNTAIN ASH – berries)

Winter

Aucuba japonica 'Crotonifolia' (SPOTTED LAUREL)
Cornus stolonifera 'Flaviramea' (DOGWOOD – stems)
Hamamelis mollis (WITCH HAZEL)
Hedera colchica 'Sulphur Heart' (PERSIAN IVY)
Ilex x altaclerensis 'Golden King' (HOLLY – berries)
Jasminum nudiflorum (WINTER JASMINE)
Mahonia x media 'Charity' (OREGON GRAPE)
Salix alba subsp. *vitellina* (WILLOW – bark)
Salvia officinalis 'Icterina' (GOLDEN SAGE)
Thymus x citriodorus 'Aureus' (GOLDEN THYME)

Green for growth

BELOW This composition sets the frothy lime-green flowers of *Alchemilla mollis* and spiky upright foliage of iris against the larger leaves of *Rheum palmatum*, *Ligularia dentata* 'Desdemona' and *Gunnera manicata*. Some contrasting red plants or accessories are all that is needed to complete the scene.

Green is the colour of nature, a balanced hue which is neither warming nor cooling and brings harmony to all in its presence. The greenness of young seedlings is a powerful image in all societies and represents regeneration and fertility. For this reason, green is believed to bring about change, create new routes in life and encourage hope. Restful and relaxing, it offers sanctuary from the outside world and engenders a feeling of peace. It is appropriate for meditation as it encourages a purposeful state of mind. In excess, however, green may slow down movement and lead to indecision.

Often preferred by the civilized and conventional who are well adjusted, it is rejected by the lonely or those with a degree of mental disturbance.

Green acts as a general tonic and detoxifier, balancing all the energies of body, mind and spirit, soothing muscles, stabilizing nerves and relieving mental stress. It is useful in the treatment of claustrophobia and its calming influence soothes headaches and controls blood pressure and nerves; it may be used to good effect with hyperactive children.

Green governs the heart chakra, the energy centre in the body that represents the chest, shoulders and lower lungs. It is therefore used to treat ailments of the heart – both physical, such as angina, and emotional. It can help to dispel negative feelings and calm and cool the emotions.

The following conditions may also respond to treatment with green: bingeing, colds, gout, hepatitis, jaundice and other liver complaints, cancer and Parkinson's disease (only in conjunction with conventional medicine), shingles, stomach problems (including ulcers, indigestion, nausea, travel sickness), thrush.

Green in the garden

The colour of the plant kingdom and the natural world, green is a very variable hue with many associations. Pale citrus greens denote the early growth of spring; deeper blue-greens are colder; brownish-greens relate to the colours of late summer and autumn. In the garden, green appears to enlarge space and will have a calming influence. It also enhances appetite and so is a useful colour for dining areas. In colour healing, green allays anxiety and brings a sense of peace and well-being. What better way can there be to engender tranquillity than communing with the growing plants in our gardens?

Although green is rarely found in natural building materials, green wood stains can be used on fences or other structures to provide an attractive backdrop. It is a popular colour for garden furniture and parasols. You may also include green glazed pots and garden ornaments.

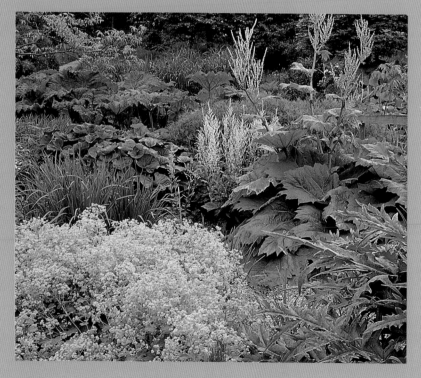

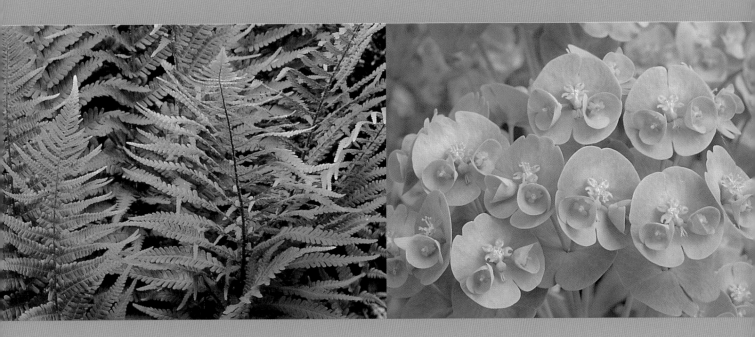

Green plants Complementary colour: red

Obviously most garden plants will be suitable for this section because of their foliage; a few of the plants listed below also produce green flowers. If you wish to use a plant which you consider suitable but which produces brightly coloured flowers at some stage, simply cut them off to retain the essential 'greenness'.

LEFT The fronds of the ostrich feather fern (*Matteucia struthiopteris*) remain a rich green throughout the summer when grown in light shade and a damp soil.

RIGHT The lime-green flowering bracts of spurge (*Euphorbia amygdaloides* var. *robbiae*) brighten the darkest corner of the garden from late winter.

Spring

Crambe cordifolia
Daphne laureola (flowers)
Helleborus argutifolius (HELLEBORE – flowers)
Hosta 'Royal Standard' (PLANTAIN LILY)
Pinus mugo (PINE)
Polystichum setiferum (SOFT SHIELD FERN)
Ribes alpinum (FLOWERING CURRANT – flowers)
Robinia pseudoacacia (FALSE ACACIA)
Viburnum davidii
Vinca minor (LESSER PERIWINKLE)

Summer

Alchemilla mollis (LADY'S MANTLE – flowers)
Angelica archangelica (ANGELICA – flowers)
Berberis thunbergii (BARBERRY)
Betula pendula (SILVER BIRCH)
Cotinus coggygria (SMOKE BUSH)
Hosta fortunei (PLANTAIN LILY)
Juniperus scopulorum 'Skyrocket' (JUNIPER)
Miscanthus sinensis 'Gracillimus'
Rosa 'Green Ice' (ROSE – flowers)
Sorbus aria (WHITEBEAM)

Autumn

Arbutus unedo (STRAWBERRY TREE)
Aucuba japonica (LAUREL)
Ballota pseudodictamnus
Buxus sempervirens 'Suffruticosa' (DWARF BOX)
Dryopteris filix-mas (MALE FERN)
Hebe cupressoides (SHRUBBY VERONICA)
Ilex aquifolium 'J C Van Tol' (HOLLY)
Itea ilicifolia (flowers)
Pterocarya fraxinifolia (CAUCASIAN WING NUT – flowers)
Yucca gloriosa

Winter

Euphorbia amygdaloides var. robbiae (SPURGE – flowers)
Fargesia murieliae (BAMBOO)
Fatsia japonica (CASTOR OIL PLANT)
Garrya elliptica
Hedera colchica (PERSIAN IVY)
Juniperus communis 'Hibernica' (IRISH JUNIPER)
Osmanthus decorus
Pachysandra terminalis
Phormium tenax (NEW ZEALAND FLAX)
Prunus laurocerasus 'Otto Luyken' (CHERRY LAUREL)

Blue for the spirit

Blue is an ideal colour for places of healing, since it encourages relaxation and tranquillity. It is a good colour for contemplation and is very conducive to meditation, inspiring patience and calm thought. Blue makes you aware of the need for rest and allows you to make space in your life. It denotes a desire for peace and order and is the colour of the present time – the Age of Aquarius.

Blue is often the first choice in colour preference tests and tends to be chosen by conservative, accomplished, deliberate and successful people. It is often rejected by those who are anxious or harbour a sense of failure.

Although very variable, it is always a cold hue and has a cooling and cleansing effect which quiets the mind and soul. Tests have shown that exposure to blue has a calming influence which reduces blood pressure, pulse rate and brainwave activity – interestingly, this is also noticeable with exposure to violet (which combines blue and red). Blue is the colour for modern-day stress and anxiety; its calming influence will relieve insomnia and combat nervousness, tension or fear. It encourages exhalation and so is very helpful in cases of asthma where it can ease symptoms of breathlessness. Inflammation and fever will be cooled and heart palpitations eased in its presence.

Blue represents the throat chakra, the energy centre within the body that is linked to the throat, upper lungs, arms and base of the skull. It is useful in the treatment of conditions such as overactive thyroid, hiccups, stuttering, gum problems, stiff necks, sore throats, tonsillitis and, particularly, childhood ailments such as teething or speech problems. Some stomach conditions may also be alleviated, including colic, colitis and stomach ulcers.

Blue in the garden

Characteristic of spring, blue brings to mind clear skies and engenders a feeling of spaciousness. It will increase the perceived space in a garden but because it does not define dimensions or set limits it requires careful placement. A wonderful colour to de-stress, it is perhaps too calming to be suitable for dining or entertainment areas.

Typical spring flowers include forget-me-nots, bluebells and bulbs such as hyacinths. However, pure blue flowers are rare in nature and the hues are variable, ranging from pale sky blues, through cool greeny-blues to richer violet-blues.

Many garden materials are available in tones of blue: granite setts are often a deep blue-grey, blue engineering bricks and pavers are common garden elements and slate paving is slightly more unusual but equally suitable. There are some wonderful ceramics with vivid blue glazes and blue is also popular for outdoor furniture and accessories such as garden chairs and parasols.

Blue plants Complementary colour: orange

There are many blue plants which provide added colour on a seasonal basis, including pansies, lobelia, petunia, love-in-the-mist, Swan River daisy, larkspur, morning glory. Besides those listed for their flowers, many plants, such as hostas, have glaucous or bluish foliage.

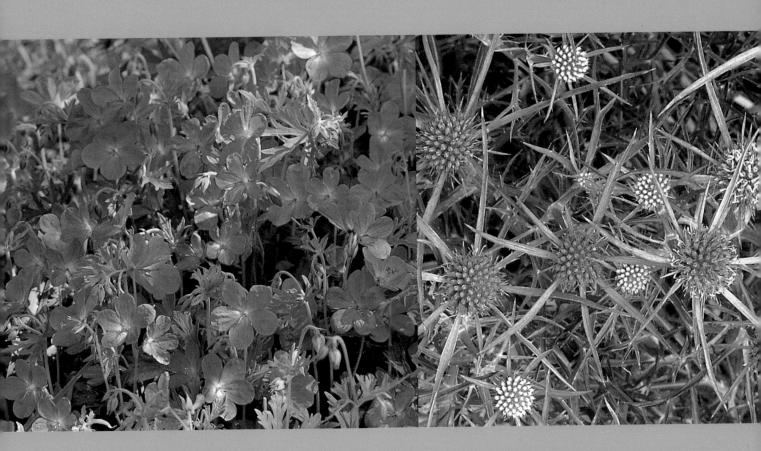

LEFT The vivid blue flowers of *Geranium* 'Johnson's Blue' provide reliable colour throughout the summer in a shade rarely found in the garden.

RIGHT As with many garden plants, it pays to hunt out selected forms to ensure the strongest hue. *Eryngium amethystinum* (sea holly) sends out clusters of thistle-like flowers in late summer and autumn.

Spring

Anemone blanda 'Atrocaerulea' (WINDFLOWER)

Aquilegia alpina (COLUMBINE)

Brunnera macrophylla

Ceanothus impressus (CALIFORNIAN LILAC)

Clematis alpina

Muscari armeniacum (GRAPE HYACINTH)

Myosotis alpestris (FORGET-ME-NOT)

Pulmonaria angustifolia 'Munstead Blue' (LUNGWORT)

Rosmarinus officinalis (ROSEMARY)

Vinca minor (LESSER PERIWINKLE)

Summer

Anchusa azurea 'Loddon Royalist'

Caryopteris x clandonensis

Ceanothus x veitchianus (CALIFORNIAN LILAC)

Delphinium hybrids

Hosta sieboldiana var. *elegans* (PLANTAIN LILY – foliage)

Iris sibirica (SIBERIAN IRIS)

Meconopsis betonicifolia (HIMALAYAN POPPY)

Nepeta x faassenii (CATMINT)

Solanum crispum 'Glasnevin' (POTATO VINE)

Teucrium fruticans (GERMANDER)

Autumn

Agapanthus campanulatus (AFRICAN LILY)

Aster x frikartii 'Monch' (MICHAELMAS DAISY)

Buddleja davidii 'Empire Blue' (BUTTERFLY BUSH)

Ceanothus x delileanus 'Gloire de Versailles' (CALIFORNIAN LILAC)

Clematis heracleifolia

Echinops ritro (GLOBE THISTLE– flowers, foliage)

Hibiscus syriacus 'Blue Bird'

Hydrangea macrophylla 'Blue Wave'

Mahonia aquifolium (OREGON GRAPE – berries)

Perovskia atriplicifolia 'Blue Spire' (RUSSIAN SAGE)

Winter

Acaena saccaticupula 'Blue Haze' (NEW ZEALAND BURR – foliage)

Chionodoxa luciliae (GLORY OF THE SNOW)

Crocus 'Blue Pearl'

Eucalyptus gunnii (GUM TREE – foliage)

Festuca glauca (BLUE FESCUE – foliage)

Hebe pimeleoides 'Quicksilver' (SHRUBBY VERONICA – foliage)

Hepatica x media 'Ballardii'

Iris reticulata

Picea pungens 'Koster' (SPRUCE – foliage)

Ruta graveolens 'Jackman's Blue' (RUE – foliage)

Violet for inner calm

Violet is a rich, regal colour which has been used throughout history to indicate knowledge, self-respect, spirituality, nostalgia, dignity and wealth. Violet brings feelings of self-worth and is a good colour to use if you need to learn to love yourself.

Not generally a popular colour, it tends to be preferred by temperamental or sensitive people with a liking for the arts and philosophical debate. A preference for violet may also be held by someone hoping to fulfil their inner desires. It is often disliked by people who hate pretence and by those who avoid close relationships.

Violet is the colour of the brow or crown chakra, the energy centre within the body that is closely linked to the 'third eye', which is said to be the centre of creative visualization. It is, therefore, a useful colour for gaining inspiration or insight into oneself and is said to enhance psychic perception; it is very conducive to meditation. It contains a potent yet balanced vibrational energy which can purify thoughts and feelings; creative people often relate well to violet and find inspiration through it.

Since it is linked to the head, colour therapists use violet to treat a range of mental disorders such as schizophrenia, the early stages of Alzheimer's disease, and concussion. It may also ease such conditions as sciatica, skin eruptions, tired or sore eyes, complaints of the nervous system, and scalp problems including dandruff. Violet also induces sleep, calms a jangled nervous system, placates emotional upset and may be used to subdue heart palpitations. It does, however, need to be handled with care as in excess it can be depressing or lead to feelings of isolation. It should not be used if there is a history of depression, nor in the treatment of young children.

With the shortest wavelength in the spectrum, beyond it lies only ultraviolet, which the human eye cannot see. Ultraviolet light is, however, detected by many insects. Some flowers have developed special patterns which are visible only under ultraviolet light, in order to entice pollinating insects.

Violet in the garden

A difficult colour to use in the garden, violet has a tendency to appear dull unless there is plenty of contrast in texture, form and tone. The softer tints of mauves and lilacs can be very restful but care needs to be taken as they can become weaker *en masse*. To lift the overall effect, include plenty of stronger tones such as that of *Berberis thunbergii* 'Atropurpurea' and make use of the strong architectural outlines of structural plants like *Phormium tenax* 'Purpureum'.

Violet is a hue rarely found in garden elements and can be a problem to accessorize. The options are probably limited to glazed pots and perhaps suitably dyed fabrics used on garden furniture.

Violet plants Complementary colour: yellow

A number of annuals can provide seasonal highlights, including pansies, petunia, ageratum, larkspur, verbena, sweet peas. The plants listed are mainly of interest for their flowers, but some have striking, purple-hued leaves.

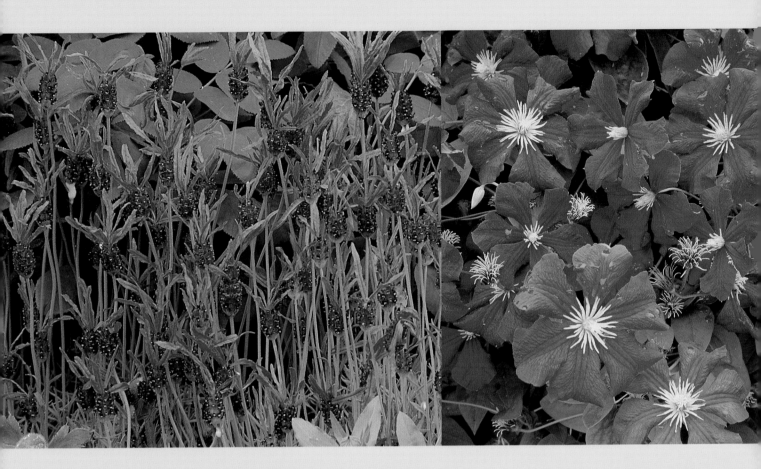

LEFT The unusual violet flowers of French lavender (*Lavandula stoechas*) contrast beautifully with the silvery foliage in summer.

RIGHT Late summer and autumn colour is provided by *Clematis viticella* 'Etoile Violette', a vigorous climber with strong purple flowers and attractive cream anthers.

Spring

Aubrieta 'J S Baker'
Cercis siliquastrum (JUDAS TREE)
Corylus maxima 'Purpurea' (PURPLE HAZEL)
Magnolia liliiflora 'Nigra'
Primula denticulata (DRUMSTICK PRIMULA)
Rhododendron 'Sleepy'
Syringa vulgaris 'Katherine Havemeyer' (LILAC)
Vinca minor 'Atropurpurea' (LESSER PERIWINKLE)
Viola labradorica 'Purpurea' (VIOLET)
Wisteria sinensis (CHINESE WISTERIA)

Summer

Allium aflatunense (ORNAMENTAL ONION)
Cistus x purpureus (SUN ROSE)
Clematis 'The President'
Delphinium 'Bruce'
Erysimum 'Bowles Mauve' (PERENNIAL WALLFLOWER)
Heuchera micrantha 'Palace Purple'
Lavandula stoechas (FRENCH LAVENDER)
Rosa 'Veilchenblau' (ROSE)
Thalictrum aquilegiifolium (MEADOW RUE)
Weigela florida 'Foliis Purpureis'

Autumn

Acanthus mollis latifolius (BEAR'S BREECHES)
Aster amellus 'King George'
Buddleja davidii 'Nanho Purple' (BUTTERFLY BUSH)
Colchicum autumnale (AUTUMN CROCUS)
Hydrangea aspera subsp. *sargentiana*
Liriope muscari (TURF LILY)
Penstemon 'Sour Grapes'
Verbena bonariensis
Viburnum plicatum 'Lanarth' (foliage)
Vitis vinifera 'Purpurea' (GRAPE VINE – foliage)

Winter

Berberis wallichiana (PURPLE BARBERRY – foliage)
Callicarpa bodinieri var. *giraldii* (berries)
Crocus chrysanthus 'Ladykiller'
Daphne mezereum (MEZEREON)
Erica carnea 'Heathwood' (HEATH)
Euonymus fortunei 'Coloratus' (foliage)
Juniperus horizontalis 'Douglasii' (JUNIPER – foliage)
Phormium tenax 'Purpureum' (NEW ZEALAND FLAX – foliage)
Rhododendron 'Blue Peter'
Salvia officinalis 'Purpurascens' (PURPLE SAGE)

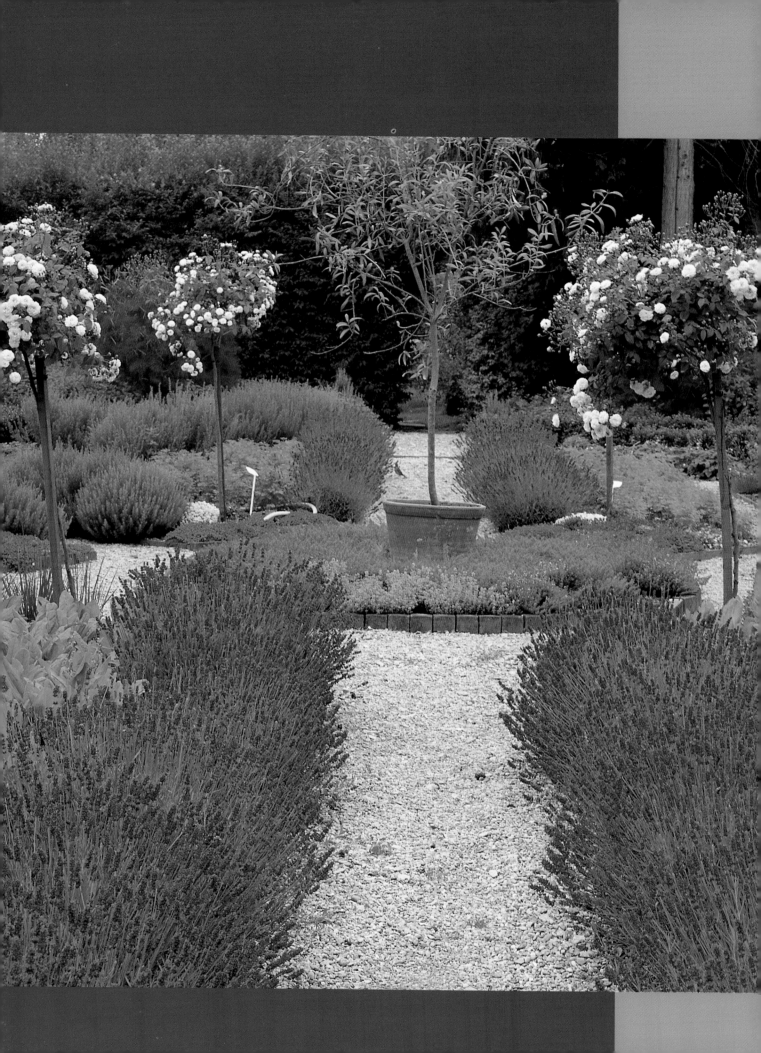

Herbalism

There is no true healing unless there is a change in outlook, peace of mind, and inner happiness.

EDWARD BACH

For thousands of years, plants have been used for the benefit of human-kind: as food, flavouring or preservative, as medicine, cosmetic, scent or dye. Within some cultures, practically every plant is considered to have useful properties and those deemed to have healing powers are particularly valued. However, the Western definition of 'herbs' has become far more compartmentalized and tends to include only those plants that we eat. This chapter offers up a selection of plants which are known to benefit health and is intended to stimulate a deeper interest in what many might consider to be ornamental garden plants.

A brief history of herbalism

The practice of 'herbalism' has evolved gradually as herbal knowledge has been passed down through generations. There are now innumerable branches of herbal medicine, yet there are often striking similarities between the principles adopted by traditional cultures throughout the world. In many of the societies where herbalism is practised today, it is believed that energy levels within the body must be in harmony or illness will ensue. Herbs are often prescribed to restore balance.

In Europe, much of the early herbal knowledge was collated from the Egyptian, Chinese and Arab nations by the ancient Greeks and Romans. They closely studied plants and used many herbs for cooking, basic hygiene and their remedial powers. They wrote up their findings in herbals – books describing the properties of plants.

Much knowledge was lost during the Dark Ages, although many traditions were preserved within the vast religious communities, and the first medicinal gardens were built in monasteries, usually alongside the infirmary.

Fortunately, herbalism continued to be practised openly throughout the Middle East, and much of the knowledge was brought back by the crusaders returning in the eleventh, twelfth and thirteenth centuries. The use of herbals developed in Europe throughout the Middle Ages, citing herbal lore alongside elements of astrology and superstition. As ever more exotic species were brought in via the new trade routes, more was written to include these previously unknown plants.

In the sixteenth and seventeenth centuries there was a widespread belief that

LEFT This ornamental herb garden demonstrates just how attractive such an area can be. Lavender hedges subdivide the garden and radiate out from a central bed which contains a potted olive tree; standard roses provide height and summer colour. It would be easy to scale these ideas up or down to suit practically any size of garden.

all plants had been put on earth for their healing benefits and it was simply a matter of matching the plant to the disorder. The sixteenth-century Doctrine of Signatures expounded the principle that plants should be prescribed according to their physical similarity to the disease being treated. For instance, the spotted leaves of *Pulmonaria officinalis* were believed to resemble the lungs and the plant was therefore often used to treat respiratory conditions, hence its common name, lungwort. Interestingly, many of these original theories have, this century, been proven to have some scientific basis.

At this time, herbs (in the widest sense of the word) were grown in 'physick' gardens where scholars could study their qualities and apothecaries would gather them for use in treatments. Plants with similar properties or of a particular type were grown together in the same bed for ease of reference and harvest. Some of the most important work of the mid seventeenth century was carried out by Nicholas Culpeper, whose detailed research into the healing powers of plants was published in his *Herbal*.

With the dawn of the scientific age and the associated development of such studies as anatomy, physiology and chemistry, botany became a true science and herbal medicine was separated from its more mystical side. Herbals now aimed to demonstrate scientific fact and further research enabled the precise classification and analysis of plants. These new medical approaches and sciences aimed to banish supernatural concepts and brought a more logical understanding of the workings of the body, sending such beliefs as the Doctrine of Signatures into demise.

From the mid seventeenth century, herbal remedies tended to be the resort of the poor; those who could afford it preferred to be treated by the new physicians. As herbalism was rejected, allopathic medicine developed: doctors now aimed to treat the disease and not the patient. Herbal remedies were equated with old wives' tales and were (and often are) not considered 'scientific' enough. Medicine as we know it was born and its practice has continued to go from strength to strength. Herbalism was dealt

a further blow with the development of pharmacology and the ability to isolate and synthesize active ingredients from plants such as foxglove (digitalis), poppy (morphine) and willow bark (aspirin). Although these new drugs were very powerful they were not without side effects.

The use of herbs today

Since the early twentieth century, the practice of herbal medicine has gradually revived and is currently attracting a great deal of interest. This seems to be due partly to an overall inclination towards a complementary approach and partly to the waning popularity of conventional medicine, no doubt connected with concerns about the side effects associated with many modern drugs. There are also many instances of herbal medicine succeeding where conventional methods have failed. Of equal importance, herbs are highly accessible and they allow us to take some control of our own well-being. Herbs work with the immune, nervous and endocrine systems to help the body adapt to the stresses of everyday life – something we all need a little help with these days.

Herbalists use all kinds of herbal material and treatments derive from every part of a plant: roots, flowers, leaves or bark. The extract is used in its entirety and contains a complex mix of constituents, bringing into play the concept of synergy: the effect of the constituents working together is more potent than the sum of their individual effects. The use of undoctored material also has a protective value as each of the elements acts as a buffer to the actions of the others. This highly complex mechanism is yet to be replicated by synthetic drugs.

As in almost every area of complementary medicine, some remedies have proven results in trials but many have not. Ask any practitioner and they will tell you that they don't necessarily know how it works...but it does! It is perhaps worth remembering that many of the treatments have been successfully used for thousands of years and that more than 60% of the world's population relies solely on herbal medicine. In fact, until the past few decades, plant-based products have been used to treat almost all disease, whether minor or life-threatening. Although, in Western society, herbalism is often scorned as 'cranky', public opinion is now changing as we return to the origins of the medicine we know today.

Homeopathy

While allopathic – what we now term 'conventional' – medicine holds that symptoms result from disease and should be repressed, homeopaths maintain that symptoms stem from the body's attempts to heal itself and provide clues to the remedy required. For this reason, substances that produce the same symptoms as the disease are used, in minute doses, as cures – like is treated with like. In homeopathic remedies, although there is barely a molecule of the original plant essence left in the treatment, it is believed that it is the plant's dynamic energy pattern that actually brings about healing. If such dilute remedies can have so potent an effect, it is conceivable that the mere presence of particular plants may be enough to bring about healing without the need to use material physically for treatment. Growing in the garden, the plant's essence might signal the body to stimulate its self-healing powers.

Practitioners of homeopathy also believe that the state of body, mind and spirit affects the progress of disease and each is of equal importance if the body is to heal itself.

Application in the garden

It is worth remembering that just because a product is natural doesn't mean that it is harmless – some of the most deadly poisons, such as strychnine, are directly derived from plant material. Many herbal remedies are very potent and although a plant growing in the garden may be quite innocuous, its healing powers should be treated with respect. There should be no side effects, as you need not come into contact with the plant, but if you do experience anything strange, steer clear of it for a while.

Enjoy the plants in their natural habitat, appreciate them for the beauty of their flower, foliage or form but, unless specifically suggested, don't apply externally and certainly don't take any but the true culinary herbs internally. If you wish to make further use of any of the plants, seek advice from a qualified herbal practitioner. Never attempt to treat a serious complaint yourself and, if a minor one does not respond quickly, seek medical advice.

Using herbs in this manner, healing will take place on a vibrational rather than physiological level. Each plant has its own unique life force or 'vibration', which can act upon and join our own energy, bringing a balance to body and mind. Herbs are thus ideal for treating a vast range of minor health problems or as an aid to other (possibly orthodox) treatments. The plants in your garden are also valuable as a preventive treatment, to harmonize problems before they manifest as disease.

The ability to heal oneself relates to the immune system; strong immunity will prevent illness by stabilizing every system within the body and fighting infection. If you feel you succumb to every bug that comes around, it would make sense to choose plants that benefit the immune system as a whole so that problems can be 'nipped in the bud'.

When you decide to turn over all or part of your garden to herbs, the opportunities are limitless. Not only do they offer much in terms of healing, but herbs also make some of the best plants for sensuous gardens, since all will please the eye and many are scented and/or edible. There is a vast range of texture, from the feathery foliage of fennel or artemisia to the soft, hairy leaves of mullein and sage. Many herbs are particularly attractive to insects, bringing the gentle hum of bees into the garden.

Most of the rules which we would apply to any other form of gardening apply equally to herb gardens. Before getting carried away with the vast selection of plants which you might wish to include, give some thought, not only to their requirements, but also your own. Where your free time is limited, make good use of perennials which will give a reliable show, year after year, with minimal input. If you spend much of your leisure time in the garden you can afford to include annuals, which will require more time and effort.

Planning your herb garden

Besides the culinary herbs we use at the table, many ornamental garden plants that we no longer think of as herbs have in the past been cultivated for their medicinal value, or their myriad household uses. Nowadays they are grown for their foliage, fragrance and colour, and range from the largest tree, through hedgerow plants, shrubs, herbaceous perennials and bulbs to the smallest creeping ground cover. Your entire plot could easily become a 'herb garden', not just the corner by the back door that supports a few pots of mint and parsley.

The first step is to forget your preconceptions about herbs being an entirely separate category of plant – there are countless varieties that work wonderfully throughout the garden, although if you plan to grow herbs for culinary use only, it probably makes sense to place them close to the house for ease of use. Every garden should appeal to the senses and herbs have an important role to play. Make use of their different colours, structures and textures to create attractive arrangements in your borders, using trees and shrubs as background elements and smaller perennials and annuals to fill in the gaps.

You would be wise to adopt an organic approach when growing herbs. Obviously this is essential if you are intending to use any of the plants for treatments or culinary purposes, but their healing powers may equally be adversely affected by chemical additives.

Although 'improved' versions of many plants are available, their ancestors, possessing more subtle form and colour, are likely to offer the most potent health benefits. However, modern hybrids will have bigger flowers, brighter foliage or better growth and you may find these preferable for practical reasons; if not, choose the original species. Always buy from a specialist nursery so that you know you are getting exactly what you want.

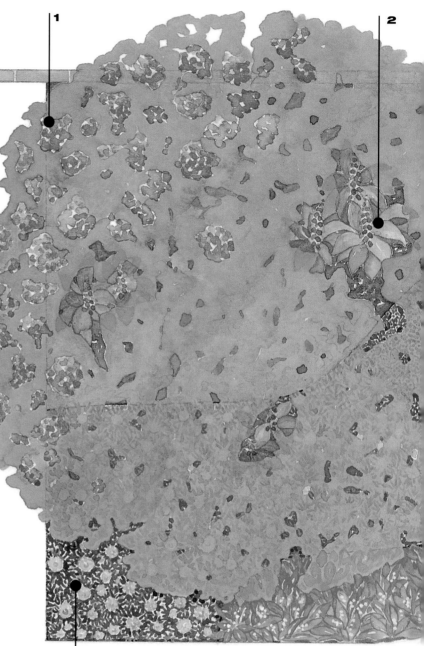

1 HAWTHORN
   (*Crataegus laevigata* 'Paul's Scarlet')

2 FOXGLOVE
   (*Digitalis purpurea*)

3 EVENING PRIMROSE
   (*Oenothera biennis*)

4 BROOM
   (*Cytisus scoparius*)

5 SWEET VIOLET
   (*Viola odorata*)

6 MILK THISTLE
   (*Silybum marianum*)

7 LILY-OF-THE-VALLEY
   (*Convallaria majalis*)

8 FALSE HELLEBORE
   (*Adonis vernalis*)

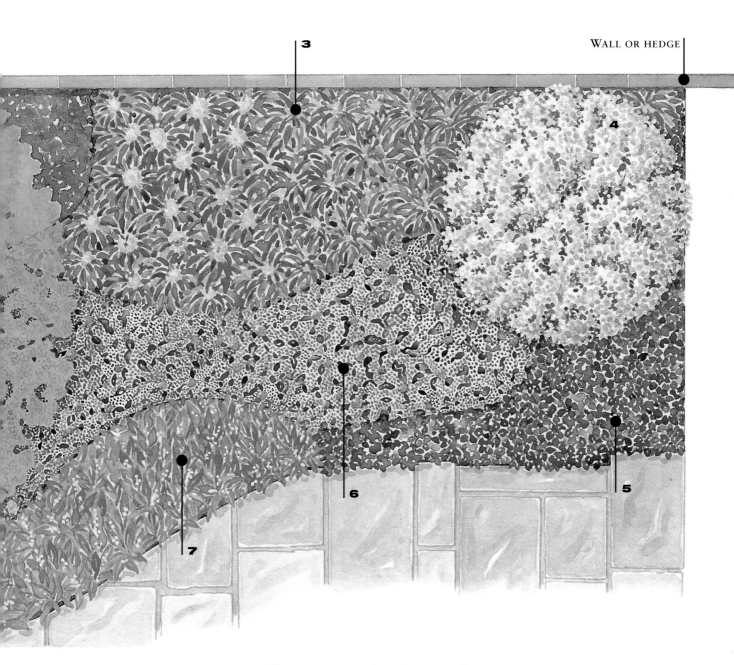

3

WALL OR HEDGE

4

6

5

7

An apothecary's border

The plants in this small, informal border have traditional links with the treatment of heart problems. The border should be fairly open, receiving sun for most of the day, with reasonably free-draining soil. Violets provide colour from very early spring, soon followed by the yellow flowers of the false hellebore and broom, and the red blossom of the hawthorn. The delicious scent of lily-of-the-valley, yellow flowers of evening primrose and marbled leaves and pink flowers of milk thistle add interest later in the year.

RIGHT Formal knot gardens epitomize the later medieval period of garden history; geometric patterns were built up using low clipped hedges, flowering bulbs and herbs. Here, box (*Buxus sempervirens*) is used but cotton lavender (*Santolina* spp.), germander (*Teucrium fruticans*) or lavender (*Lavandula* spp.) would be equally suitable.

Herbal habitats

Spend a little time planning the area before committing to any planting – take note of all the usual issues such as available space, aspect, light and shade, climate and soil conditions. Although existing conditions can be altered a little by perhaps cutting down a tree, incorporating gravel or laying drainage, such actions are not to be recommended in the main. Aim to work with nature wherever you can and select plants to suit your conditions rather than trying to alter the entire ecology of your garden.

Plants from the same ecological niche in the wild will require similar conditions and should therefore be grouped together in a spot which will suit them. Not only will this lead to healthier and stronger growth, but if allowed to grow happily and self-seed, plants will also require the minimum of maintenance.

There is a space in every garden for herbal plants. Many grow happily in full shade (Oregon grape, acanthus, periwinkle, lungwort, birth root); a few prefer light shade (bugle, foxglove, Christmas rose, betony, black cohosh); some need full sun (poppies, evening primrose, cotton lavender, pot marigold, heartsease). Damp sites or open water suit water lilies, meadowsweet, elecampane, Joe Pye weed and valerian, while pasque flowers, mullein, hyssop, Californian poppy and Scot's pine thrive in dry soil. Others are happy to grow almost anywhere (although they might be defined by some as weeds!).

Some herbs will thrive in particularly poor, thin soils and these tend to be those from the Mediterranean or similar areas; they include lavender, thyme and sage. Others, for instance parsley, chives and foxgloves, need a richer, more retentive soil to encourage lush growth. If growing herbs in containers, aim to provide the right conditions, using soil-based composts to improve water and nutrient retention or adding grit to improve drainage.

The range of habitats is almost as diverse as the number of plants:

- fill a sunny border with herbs of Mediterranean origin, which often have grey or silver foliage (artemisia, sage, santolina, verbascum)
- plant herbs (chamomile, thymes) as an alternative lawn for small areas (see page 33)
- use plants as edgings or low hedges all around the garden (lavender, chives, lady's mantle)
- create a small woodland or hedgerow habitat with dappled shade (foxgloves, primroses, silver birch, sweet woodruff)
- use climbing varieties to cover a wall or trellis (vine, passion flower, honeysuckle)
- make a pond to attract wildlife and plant herbs in or around it (water lily, meadowsweet, bog bean, purple loosestrife – see page 29)
- plant a rockery or scree garden with herbs that prefer good drainage (rock rose, thyme, sage, California poppy, mullein)
- some herbal plants are to be found growing in walls or through cracks in paving (thyme, valerian, rock rose, pennyroyal)
- a few are ideally suited to pots, hanging baskets or windowboxes, either for improved drainage or to control their growth (basil, mint, parsley, thyme, marigold).

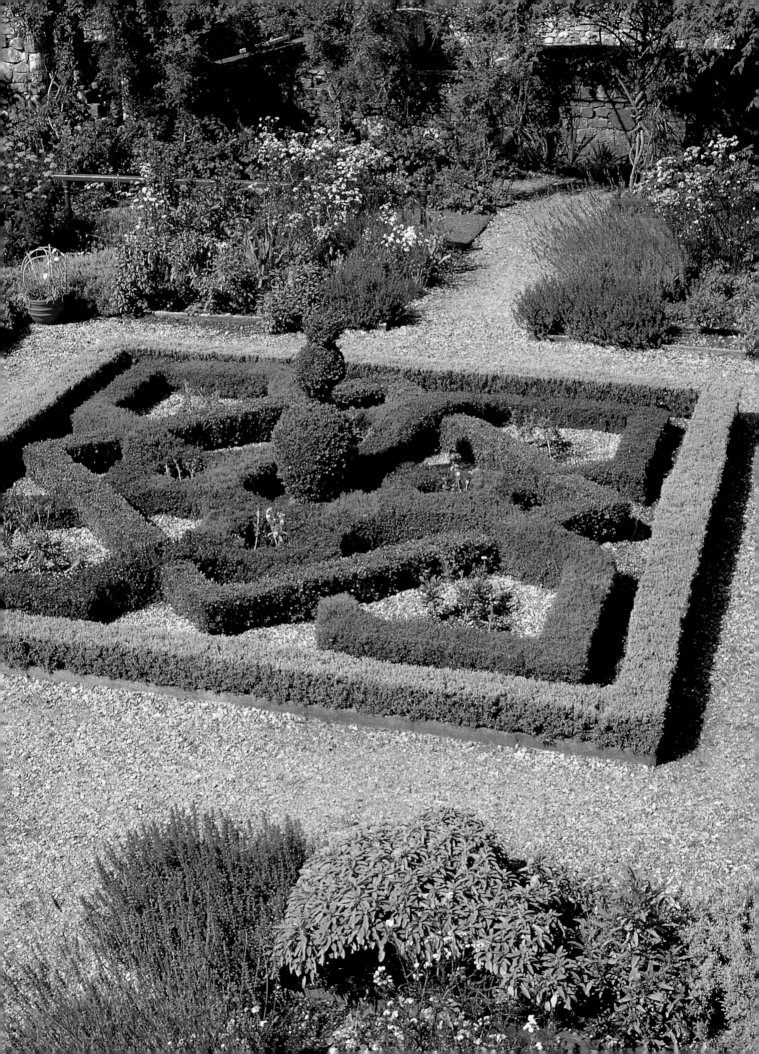

Shapes and themes

Draw up your plans and plot out a few different ideas. You might choose a formal parterre or an informal cottage garden where herbs are grown mixed in with flowers and vegetables. You can even have both, contrasting lushness of growth with neatly clipped box hedges. Look at modern ideas or more traditional approaches – whichever best suits you and your home.

Paths are important for easy access so that you can get into close contact with every plant should you so wish. Make paths attractive as well as practical; use gravel, brick, tiles or slabs to construct dry routes through the area so that you can get to the plants even after rain. Include a seat wherever possible so that you can spend time among the plants, absorbing their beneficial essence, particularly if you are using the area for convalescence. Surround the seat with plants which are particularly tactile or which need to be crushed to release their fragrance; you might even build a turf seat furnished with chamomile or thyme.

Many formal gardens contain a central feature such as a sundial, birdbath, fountain or beehive (the last being ideally placed for nectar) and in any garden you should aim to add some height with arches or screens and perhaps standard shrub roses or clipped bay, myrtle etc.

Give some thought to the placement of individual plants. Should they be positioned beneath a window where their scent will waft upwards into the house? Some may need to be crushed underfoot to release their scent, others grown in raised beds where their beauty can be admired at close quarters; a few require the support of an arbour or arch.

Although herbs are perfectly at home grown among other plants, you may wish to set aside a specific part of the garden for their growth. Such areas are often very successful when put together with a particular theme in mind (if only to limit the choice of plants to a more manageable number!). The possibilities are endless:

- a formal garden in the shape of a cartwheel, chequerboard or knot garden; such divisions are useful so that varieties can be easily found

- a kitchen garden or potager where herbs and vegetables are grown together with low edgings of chives, parsley or dwarf box (this provides ideal opportunities for companion planting, see page 18)
- a wildflower meadow (commercial seed mixtures are readily available) including daisies, heartsease, corn poppies and cowslips (see also page 23)
- a winter garden, to provide interesting shapes, colours, textures and scents: include poppy and fennel for their seedheads, snowdrops, daphne, Christmas rose or witch hazel
- a medicinal or apothecary's garden, in which particular ailments are covered by separate beds: for example digestive (wormwood, marigold, marsh mallow), respiratory (hyssop, catnip, lungwort), insomnia (betony, hawthorn, Californian poppy)
- an astrological garden; the seventeenth-century herbalist Nicholas Culpeper linked many herbs specifically to signs of the zodiac
- an eastern Paradise garden using traditional elements of Persian design such as pavilions, water, geometric shapes (passion flower, myrtle, roses, lavender, thyme, pinks, lilies)
- a historically accurate garden using only those herbs appropriate to, for example, Medieval, Tudor or Elizabethan times
- a Shakespearean garden, using herbs mentioned by the bard (primrose, bay, borage, violets, columbine)
- a children's herb garden, including herbs with a fun element, bright colours, interesting textures and edible plants (daisies, impatiens, sunflowers, marigold, nasturtium, violets, lemon balm)
- a Chinese herb garden (opium poppy, black bamboo, *Rosa chinensis*, ginkgo, peony)
- a garden that includes only plants found naturally in your region; this will make for a particularly rich wildlife habitat
- a garden to ward off evil influences (Christmas rose, elder, crab apple, chamomile, lovage, St John's wort).

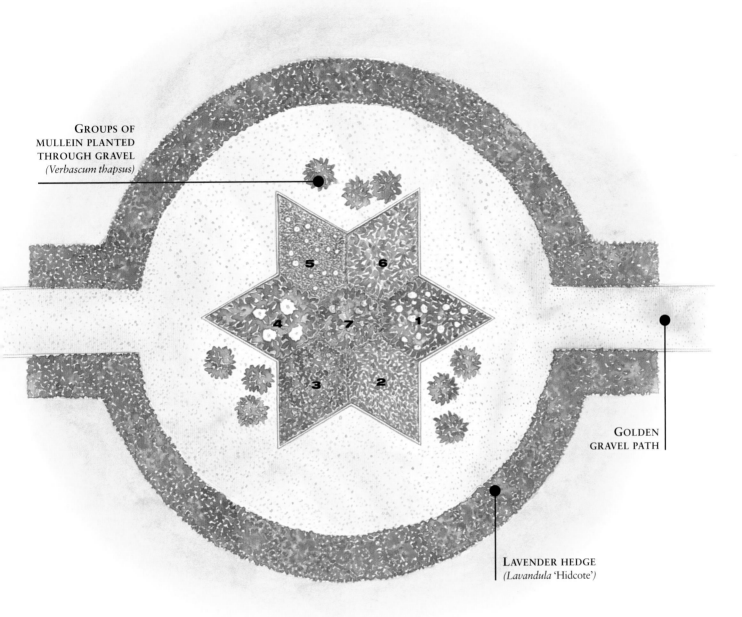

GROUPS OF
MULLEIN PLANTED
THROUGH GRAVEL
(Verbascum thapsus)

GOLDEN
GRAVEL PATH

LAVENDER HEDGE
(Lavandula 'Hidcote'*)*

1 CHRISTMAS ROSE
(Helleborus niger)

2 VERVAIN
(Verbena officinalis)

3 HEARTSEASE
(Viola tricolor)

4 PEONY
(Paeonia lactiflora)

5 CHAMOMILE
(Chamaemelum nobile)

6 ANGELICA
(Angelica archangelica)

7 ST JOHN'S WORT
(Hypericum perforatum)

A garden to ward off evil spirits

The six-pointed star is a powerful ancient symbol; in this planting it encloses seven plants, traditionally a lucky number. The groups of mullein and the lavender hedge bring the total number of plants to nine, another number once held sacred. The St John's wort in the centre provides the golden colour of the sun, symbolizing the life force of daylight. The plants have been chosen to provide colour and interest throughout the year and all are suitable for an open, well-drained site sheltered from strong winds.

Culinary herbs

There can be few greater yet more simple pleasures than picking fresh herbs from the garden to enhance the flavour of your food. It is so satisfying to be able to pick them as you need them, when their flavour is at its best, and not have to rely on dried substitutes. Most also have beneficial health properties, many of which relate directly to digestion.

The herbs you plant will reflect your personal tastes, but may also be guided by the site or available space. The following list includes the most popular culinary herbs and a few that are rarely sold in supermarkets but that are nonetheless very rewarding to grow and delicious to eat.

Allium schoenoprasum (CHIVES)
Perennial bulb to 20cm with narrow, pungent foliage and spherical, purplish flower heads in summer. Grows in sun or partial shade; prefers rich soil. As a companion plant, deters aphids.
Leaves and flowers have a mild onion flavour. Use in salads and soups, and as a garnish.
Stimulates the appetite and aids digestion. Mild antibiotic.

Aloysia triphylla (LEMON VERBENA)
Half hardy perennial to 1.2m with shiny yellow-green leaves and tiny lavender flowers in late summer. Prefers full sun and a sheltered position, and light, well-drained soil. The leaves release a strong lemon scent when crushed or chopped; dried leaves retain the scent.
Excellent in potpourri. Use in drinks, ice creams and puddings or infuse as a herb tea.
Mild sedative. Relieves nasal and bronchial congestion. Reduces indigestion and nausea.

Anethum graveolens (DILL)
Annual to 1m with feathery, aromatic, blue-green foliage and umbels of small yellow flowers in midsummer. Prefers full sun and free-draining soil.
The leaves are used to decorate and flavour cream cheese, potato salads and fish dishes. The seeds are used in both savoury and sweet dishes, or chewed to sweeten the breath.
Cures hiccups, soothes colic and indigestion; relieves nausea, flatulence and stress-related digestive disorders. Tonic for the nervous system, with sedative properties. Relieves painful periods and regulates menstruation. The oil has anti-cancer properties.

Anthriscus cerefolium (CHERVIL)
Annual to 45cm with delicate, pale green, ferny foliage and tiny white flowers through summer. Prefers light shade and well-drained soil.
Its elegant leaves are used to garnish fish and egg dishes. Their subtle flavour is best appreciated when added to a dish shortly before serving.
Stimulates digestion. Relieves catarrh. Improves circulation and helps liver complaints.

Armoracia rusticana (HORSERADISH)
Perennial to 1m with large, elliptical leaves; a variegated form is available. Prefers an open, sunny site and rich, moist soil. Makes a good companion plant to potatoes, helping to prevent disease in the tubers.
Grown mainly for its root, which is grated and mixed with vinegar, cream or mayonnaise to make a sauce for roast beef or fish – but beware, its pungent volatile oils can make your eyes water.
Stimulates digestion. Eliminates excess mucus and detoxifies. Relieves sciatica and rheumatism. A teaspoon of the grated root mixed with an equal amount of honey eases coughs and bronchitis.

Artemisia dracunculus (FRENCH TARRAGON)
Perennial to 60cm with narrow, fragrant, spicy

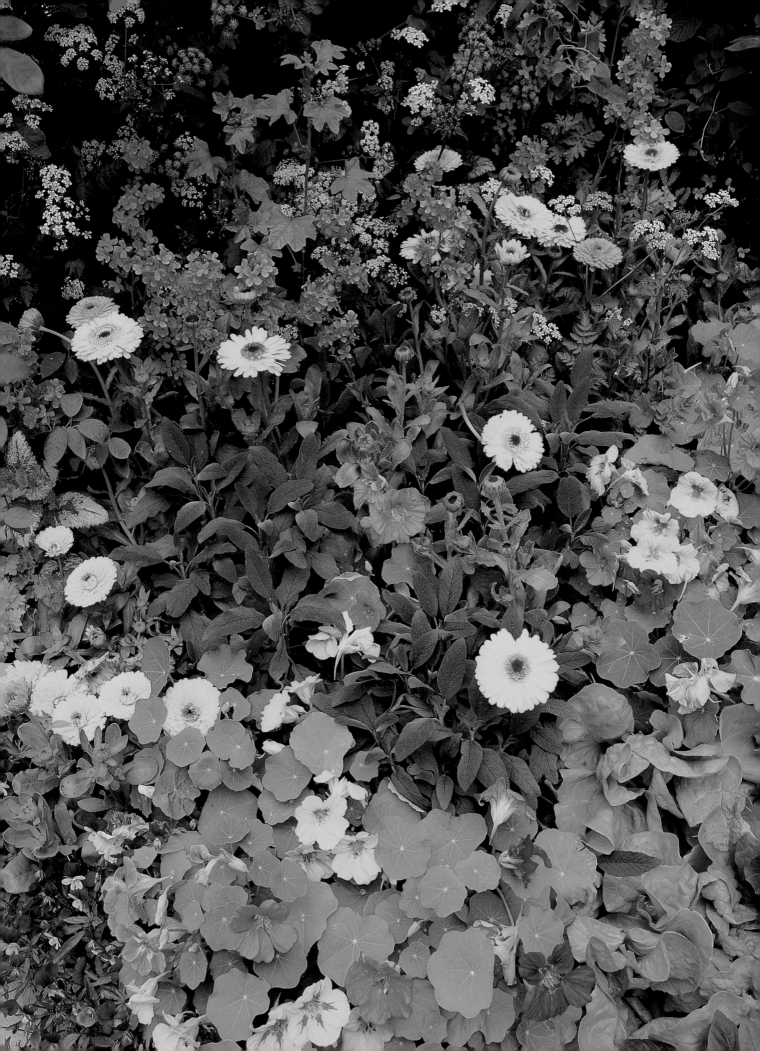

(slightly aniseed) leaves. Needs a sunny, sheltered site and rich, well-drained soil.

The leaves can be infused in vinegar for use in salad dressings. The keynote of Béarnaise sauce, tarragon is also a classic with chicken and eggs.

Rich in mineral salts, tarragon acts as a general tonic and stimulates the appetite. It has also been used to relieve toothache.

Borago officinalis (BORAGE)

Annual to 60cm with large, prickly-hairy leaves and sky-blue, star-shaped flowers in summer. Likes sun and light, well-drained soil. Attracts bees and makes a good companion plant for tomatoes and strawberries.

The flowers are used to decorate savoury dishes, fruit salads, cakes and drinks. The young leaves have a cucumber flavour and can be chopped and used in salads and sandwiches.

Relaxant; eases grief and sadness. Soothes inflammation of respiratory, digestive and urinary systems; relieves fever; diuretic. Stimulates the adrenal glands (counters the effects of steroids). Contains gamma-linoleic acid, the active ingredient in evening primrose oil, which relieves pre-menstrual syndrome, allergies, skin conditions (eczema) and arthritis/rheumatism.

Carum carvi (CARAWAY)

Biennial to 30cm with feathery foliage and umbels of tiny white flowers in midsummer. Prefers full sun and rich soil.

Grown mainly for its seeds, which are traditional with pork and cabbage dishes, in apple pie, cakes and biscuits. Kummel liqueur and some north European cheeses are flavoured with caraway, and the seeds are chewed at the end of an Indian meal to sweeten the breath.

Soothes digestive disorders; relieves flatulence and colic.

Coriandrum sativum (CORIANDER)

Hardy annual to 60cm with bright green, finely cut, fragrant foliage and umbels of small white or mauve flowers through summer. Likes full sun and rich, light soil.

The aromatic seeds are used whole or ground as a spice for many dishes. The leaves are added to soups, stews, curries and salads from central and south America and Asia; many Thai dishes also use coriander roots.

Aids digestion; reduces colic and flatulence. Mild sedative; eases rheumatic pain.

Foeniculum vulgare (FENNEL)

Hardy perennial to 2m with feathery leaves and umbels of yellow flowers in midsummer. Likes full sun and well-drained soil.

Fennel seeds and leaves are used to flavour fish dishes; in Provence, fish are grilled over dried fennel stalks. (The bulbous vegetable is a different variety of fennel.)

Gentle calming properties may alleviate stomach cramps, relieve indigestion and constipation and help to control weight gain. Also used to treat eye ailments, coughs and catarrh. Avoid when pregnant.

Hyssopus officinalis (HYSSOP)

Semi-evergreen perennial to 60cm with aromatic, dark green, narrow leaves and whorls of tiny blue flowers in summer; flowers in other colours available. Attracts bees and butterflies; good companion plant for cabbages. Prefers full sun and well-drained soil.

The flowers decorate salads. Use leaves very sparingly to flavour pâtés, pulses and stews.

Wards off infection and enhances immunity. Tonic to the nervous system – releases tension. Relieves respiratory problems; stimulates the circulation; brings down fever. Aids digestion. Avoid when pregnant.

Levistichum officinale (LOVAGE)

Herbaceous perennial to 2m with dark green, glossy, aromatic, divided foliage and umbels of yellow-green flowers in summer. Thrives in sun or partial shade and rich, moist soil.

Seeds, leaves, stems and roots are all edible, with a strong, savoury, celery-like flavour. Use in soups, stews and salads; good with chicken or in vegetarian dishes.

Aphrodisiac and stimulant; eases indigestion and bronchial congestion. Diuretic; an infusion of seeds or leaves can detoxify, reduce water retention and ease rheumatism. Avoid when pregnant or if you have kidney problems.

Melissa officinalis (LEMON BALM)

Perennial to 60cm with bright green, lemon-scented leaves and small white flowers in summer. Variegated and golden-leaved varieties available. Prefers morning sun, afternoon shade, and moist soil. Attracts bees.

Float fresh leaves in cold drinks, chop and add to fruit salads, or infuse leaves for herb tea or custard. Also good with fish and chicken.

Once known as 'cure-all', lemon balm boosts the immune system and calms the nerves. It eases stress, anxiety and depression, headaches and migraine, feverish colds and insomnia, menstrual and digestive problems, nausea and high blood pressure.

Mentha spicata (SPEARMINT)

Perennial to 60cm with strongly scented, wrinkled foliage and spikes of mauve flowers in late summer. Likes sun or partial shade and rich, moist soil. Plant as companion to roses to deter aphids.

Good with potatoes, peas and lamb. Infuse fresh or dried leaves for herb tea.

Relieves cold symptoms.

Mentha suaveolens rotundifolia (APPLE MINT)

Perennial to 60cm with hairy, apple-scented, bright green leaves and spikes of pale lilac flowers in summer; also variegated form. Prefers partial shade, rich soil.

Add to fruit salads and cold drinks.

Aids digestion. Eases colds and flu.

Ocimum basilicum (BASIL)

Tender annual to 45cm with aromatic, glossy leaves and small white flowers; varieties include purple basil and small-leaved bush basil. Requires warm sun and protection from wind and frost; well-drained, moist soil.

Leaves are widely used in Mediterranean and Asian cooking.

Calming yet uplifting effect – treats both insomnia and mental fatigue. Rub leaves on temples to relieve headaches. Infuse fresh leaves to prevent travel sickness. Reduces stress, regulates menstrual cycle, relieves muscular aches.

Origanum vulgare (OREGANO)

Perennial to 60cm with aromatic, small green leaves and clusters of fragrant pink or white flowers in summer; other varieties available including golden-leaved. Needs full sun and free-draining soil. Attracts bees and butterflies.

Use fresh or dried leaves with fish and tomato-based dishes.

Infuse as a tea to prevent seasickness, soothe coughs, stomach and gallbladder problems, nervous headaches, irritability and exhaustion. Antiseptic. Relieves rheumatism.

Petroselinum crispum (PARSLEY)

Biennial to 40cm with toothed, curled leaves; flat-leaved variety available. Prefers full sun or light shade and rich soil.

Myriad culinary uses: as a garnish, in soups and sauces.

Rich in vitamins and minerals, for general health and clear skin. Antiseptic. Breath freshener Digestive tonic. Diuretic – relieves urinary disorders, including kidney problems.

Pimpinella anisum (ANISE)

Annual to 45cm with aromatic, round, mid-green leaves and clusters of tiny white flowers in late summer. Needs a sunny, sheltered site and rich, well-drained soil.

Grown mainly for its seed, which is used to flavour cakes, confectionery, liqueurs and curries.

Antiseptic. Eases coughs and bronchitis. Soothes colic; relieves nausea.

Rosmarinus officinalis (ROSEMARY)

Evergreen shrub to 1.8m with narrow leathery leaves – dark green with white-felted undersides –

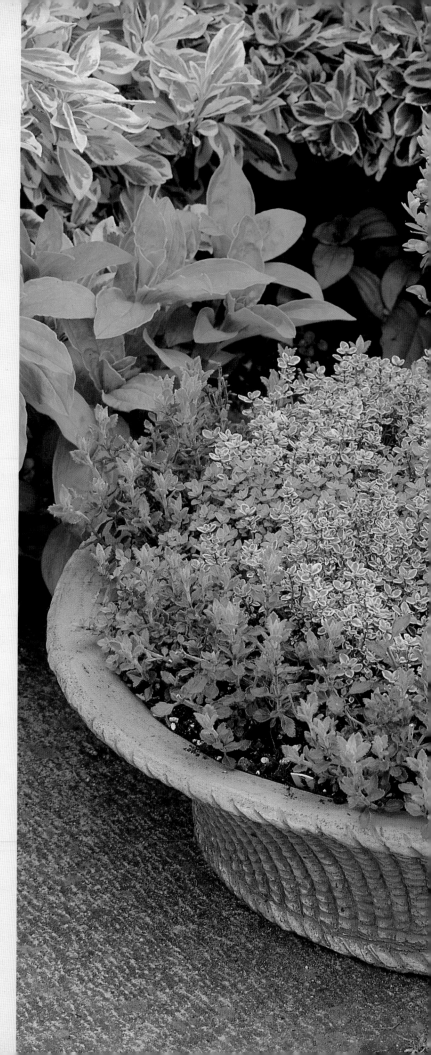

and bluish, orchid-like flowers in late spring. Needs
sun and well-drained soil.
Flavours stews and roasts, especially lamb.
Antiseptic. Improves digestion. Invigorating tonic;
strengthens nervous system and circulation – good for
high blood pressure. Relieves aches and pains,
headaches, nasal congestion. Good for skin and hair.

Salvia officinalis (SAGE)
Evergreen shrub to 75cm with hairy grey-green
leaves and purple flowers; coloured foliage varieties
also available. Prefers sun and well-drained soil.
*Mix with onion for a stuffing for chicken, goose
and pork; also good with liver.*
Antiseptic. Relieves sore throats, catarrh, bronchitis,
asthma, tuberculosis. Antioxidant properties – delays the
ageing process. Enhances immune function (AIDS).
Cleansing for arthritis and gout; beneficial to liver.
Digestive remedy – eases colic and flatulence, stimulates
the appetite. Tonic for the female reproductive system
including menopausal symptoms (contains oestrogen).
Nerve tonic for stress. Avoid when pregnant.

Satureja montana (WINTER SAVORY)
Evergreen perennial to 40cm with aromatic,
narrow, dark green leaves and spikes of white or
pale lilac flowers in summer. Prefers full sun and
well-drained soil.
Use in dishes of fresh or dried beans.
Stimulates the appetite; aids digestion; eases indigestion
and flatulence. Brings down fevers. Crush leaf and apply
to insect stings to relieve pain.

Thymus vulgaris (COMMON THYME)
Evergreen shrub with tiny, aromatic leaves and
pink or lilac flowers in summer. Attracts bees.
Prefers full sun and well-drained soil. Many forms
available, with various foliage and flower colours
and growing habits.
*Myriad culinary uses for fresh or dried leaves: in
marinades, sauces, stuffings.*
Antiseptic – for coughs, sore throats and colds. Increases
resistance to infection. Aids digestion. An infusion of fresh
leaves acts as a hangover cure. Avoid when pregnant.

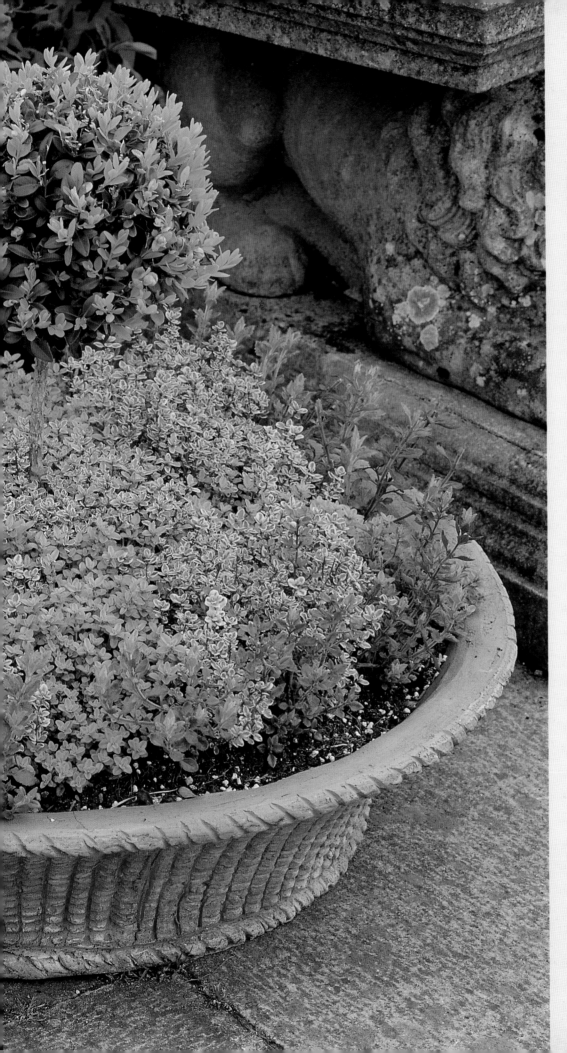

LEFT Even the tiniest
garden or balcony can
support a few herbs for
the kitchen. This shallow
terracotta bowl is
perfectly suited for the
growth of thyme; a mix,
including golden and
lemon-scented varieties
have been planted
together here. The
clipped box lollipop adds
a further dimension of
height to the composition.

Healing plants

The following plants all have healing properties but are not normally regarded as herbs. The qualities described relate to both herbal and homeopathic usage. Plants whose essential oils are used for healing (for example, yarrow, lavender, pine) will be found in the chapter on Aromatherapy.

Many wild plants – so-called 'weeds' such as dandelion and nettle – are often used in herbal treatments, but these have been omitted since most people will probably prefer not to encourage their growth within the cultivated garden. However, they do have an important role to play and you might wish to include such plants if you have the space for a wilder area.

Most of the plants listed are completely safe to include in the garden, although they should not used for specific home treatments without further advice. However, a few are poisonous; if young children use the garden it is probably wise to exclude potentially dangerous plants. Although the general advice is to avoid the use of all herbal remedies during pregnancy, plants simply grown in the garden are highly unlikely to cause any problems. However, some have specific properties relating to pregnancy and childbirth and it might be wise to avoid their inclusion in the garden at this time.

The following plant descriptions are fairly brief – once you have drawn up a shortlist of plants, refer to specialist books for further details of required growing conditions.

★ Avoid use during pregnancy

✖ Plant is or has potential to be toxic

Acanthus mollis (ACANTHUS)
Semi-evergreen perennial to 1.2 x 1m with deep green, lobed, glossy foliage and spikes of white and purple flowers in summer.
Eases strained joints and burns. Relieves problems of the digestive and urinary tracts.

Adonis vernalis (FALSE HELLEBORE) ✖
Perennial to 40 x 25cm with ferny foliage and buttercup-like, yellow flowers in early spring.

RIGHT False hellebore (*Adonis vernalis*) produces attractive bright yellow flowers in spring; the plant is used to treat a variety of conditions relating to the heart.

FAR RIGHT Bugle (*Ajuga reptans*) is a British native which assists the healing of cuts and bruises.

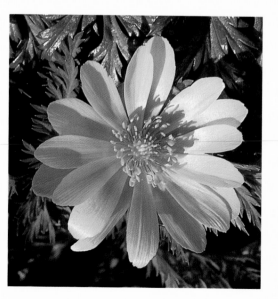

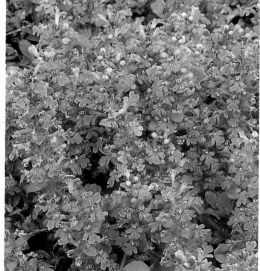

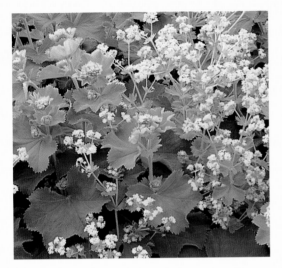

Improves heart function, relieves angina, raises blood pressure, improves circulation.

Ajuga reptans (BUGLE)
Evergreen creeping perennial to 30 x 45cm with oval leaves and spikes of deep blue flowers in early summer; coloured-leaved varieties available.
Analgesic. Heals wounds and bruises – staunches bleeding. Cleanses liver. Lowers blood pressure.

Alchemilla vulgaris (LADY'S MANTLE) ★
Herbaceous perennial to 30 x 45cm with soft green pleated leaves and greenish yellow flowers in loose panicles mid to late summer.
Relates strongly to feminine issues; relieves gynaecological problems and eases symptoms of menopause; encourages conception. Staunches blood flow, heals wounds, reduces inflammation.
Also eases all kinds of transitions in life.

Alcea rosea (HOLLYHOCK), Althaea officinalis (MARSH MALLOW)
Perennials to 2 x 1m with velvety, grey-green, lobed leaves and pale pink or white flowers in late summer.
Reduces inflammation and irritation of internal systems, including irritable bowel syndrome. Treats boils and abscesses, insect stings. Eases coughs and chest infections. Relieves insomnia.

Arnica montana (ARNICA) ✖
Aromatic perennial to 60cm with a rosette of downy leaves and golden yellow, scented, daisy-like flowers from midsummer to early autumn.
Improves resistance to infection. Improves local blood supply and speeds healing of bruises, sprains, muscle strain, concussion, gout, rheumatism. For mental and physical shock, including after a stroke; allows the sufferer to recover from trauma more easily.

Artemisia vulgaris (MUGWORT) ★
Perennial to 100 x 60cm with finely cut dark green leaves and clusters of reddish or yellow flowers.
Antiseptic. Tonic – stimulates the digestion, antispasmodic effect eases colic and indigestion. Menstrual problems of all types including menopausal; increases fertility. Treats fluid retention – eliminator and blood cleanser for gout, arthritis. Mildly sedative and beneficial to the nervous system, for epilepsy, dizziness and sleepwalking.
Also helps to 'ground' a person and balance their practical side with their emotions.

Asplenium scolopendrium (HARTSTONGUE)
Evergreen fern to 60 x 30cm with tongue-shaped, leathery, bright green fronds.
Astringent to heal wounds. Relieves diarrhoea and colitis. Benefits the liver and spleen.

Baptisia tinctoria (FALSE INDIGO) ✖
Perennial to 1.2 x 0.6m with blue-green foliage and lupin-like, yellow flowers in early summer.
Antiseptic and anti-inflammatory. Detoxifies. Stimulates the immune system. Relieves respiratory conditions.

Bellis perennis (DAISY)
Perennial lawn 'weed' to 7cm with oval, hairy leaves and pinkish white flowers through summer; also double forms.
Good remedy for children. Treats women's reproductive problems. Eases rheumatic aches and pains, bruises, general stiffness and backache. Detoxifies to relieve arthritis, gout, acne, diarrhoea, coughs and colds.
Also clears the mind and enhances concentration.

LEFT Lady's mantle (Alchemilla vulgaris) has been used for centuries for health problems relating to women; it is also used to improve the healing of wounds.

Calendula officinalis (POT MARIGOLD) ★
Annual to 60 x 60cm with pale green, hairy foliage and bright orange, daisy-like flowers in summer.
Stimulates the immune system to fight infection; also anti-cancer action. Improves circulation; fights fever; detoxifies; anti-inflammatory – for gout, arthritis. Soothes the digestive system. Antiseptic and astringent – heals external wounds and inflammation such as ulcers, varicose veins, skin problems, eczema. Beneficial to the female reproductive system; regulates menstruation.
Also engenders warmth and compassion.

Catalpa bignonioides (INDIAN BEAN TREE)
Deciduous tree to 15 x 15m with large, green leaves and spikes of white flowers in summer followed by long pods.
Sedative; eases asthma and whooping cough. Relieves eye ailments.

Centaurea cyanus (CORNFLOWER)
Annual to 90 x 60cm with narrow, grey-green leaves and double, daisy-like flowers in blues, pinks, purples, white all summer.
Raises resistance to infection. Relieves eye problems. Improves the digestion and supports the liver. Eases rheumatic complaints.

Cimicifuga racemosa (BLACK COHOSH)
Perennial to 1.5 x 0.6m with toothed foliage and long spikes of small creamy-white flowers through summer and autumn.
For nerve and muscle pain – arthritis, rheumatism, headaches, tinnitus. Antispasmodic, sedative – relieves asthma. Lowers blood pressure, normalizes heart function. Beneficial to female reproductive system, including menstruation and menopause; prepares the body for childbirth.
Also for depression in women; increases positivity.

Cnicus benedictus (BLESSED THISTLE) ★
Annual to 60 x 45cm with pale green, spiny leaves and pale yellow, thistle flowers in summer.
Tonic during convalescence, improves the nervous system. Enhances appetite and aids digestion, boosts a sluggish liver. Supports the immune system – sometimes used in cancer treatment. Antibiotic. Improves the circulation – for headaches, migraine, nerve pain, varicose veins. Eases menstrual problems, including menopausal symptoms.
Also helps you to trust your own judgement.

Colchicum autumnale (MEADOW SAFFRON) ★ ✖
Perennial corm with fleshy foliage after flowers; lilac crocus-like flowers in autumn to 30cm.
Remedy for gout, rheumatism, neuralgia and external irritation. Used in cancer research.

Convallaria majalis (LILY-OF-THE-VALLEY) ✖
Perennial bulb to 20 x 30cm with rich green foliage and drooping, white, fragrant flowers in late spring followed by red berries.
Diuretic. Reduces high blood pressure. Useful in recovery from stroke. Clears congestive conditions of the heart and emphysema.

Crataegus laevigata/C. monogyna (HAWTHORN)
Deciduous tree to 6 x 6m with thorny branches, small lobed leaves and white flowers in spring followed by red berries; other cultivars are available with double and pink or red flowers.
Heart and circulation tonic – improves poor memory by enhancing blood flow to brain, normalizes blood pressure, for hardening of the arteries, angina. Relieves stress, aids sleep.
Also for all emotional problems, including a broken heart.

Cytisus scoparius (BROOM) ★
Deciduous shrub to 2 x 2m with tiny green leaves and yellow, pea-like flowers in spring.
General tonic for the blood. Calms the heart but raises blood pressure. Diuretic – for gout. Treats the liver and kidneys, counters fluid retention.

Daphne mezereum (MEZEREON) ✖
Deciduous shrub to 1.2 x 1.2m with narrow green leaves and rosy-purple flowers in late winter followed by red berries.
Eases rheumatic joints. Improves blood flow.

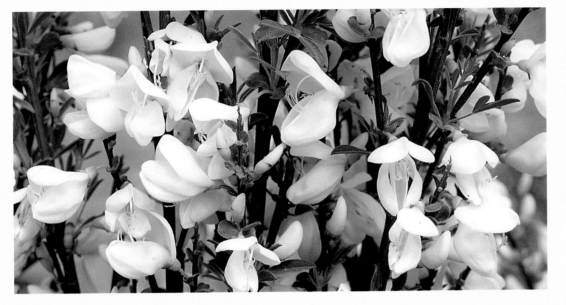

LEFT *Cytisus scoparius* 'Cornish Cream' is a selected cultivar of broom; although perhaps not as potent as the type, it may be planted for the treatment of various disorders in gardens where its softer colours are preferred.

Dictamnus albus (BURNING BUSH) ✖ ★
Perennial to 1 x 0.6m with fragrant, dark green foliage and racemes of white or pink flowers in early summer, followed by explosive seed capsules.
Antispasmodic effect on the intestinal tract. Stimulates the muscles of the uterus. Relieves nervous conditions, rheumatic pain, kidney problems. Reduces fever.

Digitalis purpurea (FOXGLOVE) ✖
Biennial growing to 1 x 0.3m with broad, downy, mid-green leaves and purple or white flowers in early summer; other colours available.
Heart tonic – used to treat weak and irregular heart rhythms, heart disease.

Echinacea purpurea (PURPLE CONEFLOWER)
Perennial to 1 x 0.5m with rough, dull green foliage and pink or purple daisy flowers with dark orange centres mid to late summer.
Currently one of the most popular herbal remedies, used to boost the immune system and fight off infection of all types such as colds and flu. Also brings down fever, treats blood poisoning, urinary infection, and is beneficial for HIV, AIDS and ME. Antibiotic and antifungal. Anti-inflammatory properties ease arthritis, gout and rheumatism. Stimulates the circulation, relieves allergies and asthma.

Also improves resilience to stress and assists recovery from trauma.

Eryngium maritimum (SEA HOLLY)
Perennial to 45 x 45cm with glaucous, spiny foliage and steely-blue, thistle-like flowers in summer.
General tonic. Diuretic – for cystitis, kidney stones. Relieves chest problems.

Eschscholzia californica (CALIFORNIAN POPPY)
Annual to 60 x 30cm with grey-green, ferny foliage and orange, yellow, cream, red or pink poppy-like flowers in summer.
Similar, but less powerful, action to *Papaver somniferum* (opium poppy). Muscle relaxant and antispasmodic for tension headaches, migraine, neuralgia. Aids sleep, relieves stress. Lowers blood pressure and heart rate, improves circulation.
Also reduces reliance upon drugs or alcohol.

Eupatorium purpureum (JOE PYE WEED)
Perennial to 2 x 1m with toothed, oval, mid-green leaves, purplish stems and heads of scented, rose-purple flowers in late summer.
Diuretic – eases urinary problems, kidney stones and cystitis. Relieves rheumatism and gout. Brings down fever (used by Native North Americans to treat typhoid).

Filipendula ulmaria (MEADOWSWEET)
Perennial to 1.2 x 0.5m with divided, wrinkled, fragrant mid-green foliage (also available in golden-leaved variety) and clusters of scented cream flowers through summer.

Soothes upset stomach, diarrhoea, irritable bowel syndrome. Sedative; soothes tension, reduces blood pressure. Relieves fever and eases rheumatic and arthritic pain, colds/flu and headaches (similar action to aspirin). Treats diabetes. Good for kidney problems.

Galium odoratum (SWEET WOODRUFF)
Perennial to 30 x 90cm with whorls of scented, bright green leaves and clusters of tiny white flowers in late spring.

Invigorates and refreshes – tonic to whole system. Softens and tones skin; anti-wrinkle possibilities. Relieves insomnia. Diuretic, anti-inflammatory, antispasmodic, anticoagulant. Treats varicose veins and wounds, relieves stomach ache.

Gaultheria procumbens (WINTERGREEN)
Evergreen shrub to 15 x 60cm with glossy, dark green leaves and pinky-white flowers in midsummer followed by red fruits.

Anti-inflammatory and antiseptic action. Relieves skin problems. Soothes the digestive system. Eases sore limbs, neuralgia, headaches and rheumatism.

Gentiana lutea (YELLOW GENTIAN) ★
Perennial to 1.5 x 0.6m with stiff, yellow-green leaves and spikes of yellow star-like flowers in late summer and autumn.

General tonic for convalescence: stimulates the appetite and tones the digestive system, improves absorption of nutrients. Detoxifier for rheumatism and gout. Brings down fever. Stimulates the female reproductive system. Not advisable during pregnancy.

Geranium maculatum (CRANESBILL)
Perennial to 60 x 60cm with lobed, mid-green, hairy leaves and pink-purple flowers in early summer.

Relieves haemorrhoids, stomach ulcers, diarrhoea, menstrual problems, irritable bowel syndrome. Also eases depression and provides motivation.

Hamamelis virginiana (WITCH HAZEL)
Deciduous shrub to 3 x 3m with coarsely toothed, oval leaves and sweetly scented yellow flowers in winter.

Treats external skin problems and speeds healing of eczema, scalds and burns, bruises, sprains, insect stings, chilblains. Staunches bleeding for nosebleeds, varicose veins. Good for female reproductive problems. Also for those under pressure of living up to the expectations of others.

RIGHT Yellow gentian (*Gentiana lutea*) produces tall flowering spikes in late summer; its primary use is related to problems with the digestive system.

FAR RIGHT The petals of some cranesbills can be added to salads, where they may assist digestive problems.

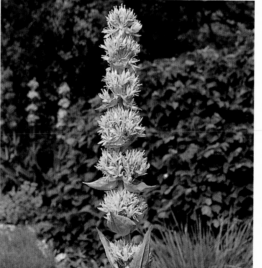

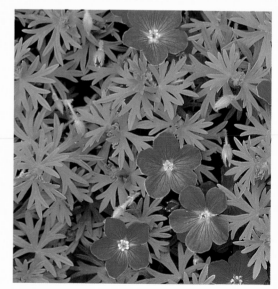

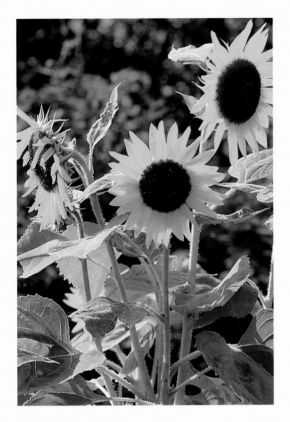

eases tension. Widely used to treat depression, imparting warmth and energy and improving positivity. Reduces symptoms of seasonal affective disorder (SAD) and hormonal changes during the menopause; eases menstrual problems including pre-menstrual syndrome. Relieves headaches, stomach cramps and internal aches and pains. Eases inflammation – cuts, burns, bruises, insect bites. Tonic for the liver and gall bladder. Relieves gout and arthritis.

Also for people who have phobias or allergies, and are oversensitive.

Inula helenium (ELECAMPANE) ★
Herbaceous perennial to 2 x 1.5m with large, light green foliage and yellow, daisy-like flowers in late summer.

Antibacterial – treats coughs, chest infections, bronchitis. Anti-inflammatory. Stimulates the immune system. Relieves allergies, including asthma. Tonic for the digestive system, improves absorption of nutrients.

Iris versicolor (BLUE FLAG) ★
Perennial to 1 x 0.6m with grey-green, lanceolate foliage and blue-violet flowers in early summer.

Enhances the immune system and lymph circulation. Purifies the blood and detoxifies, particularly the liver. Enhances the digestive system. Relieves headaches. Treats skin complaints, including acne and eczema.

Also releases creative blocks and enhances progress through life.

Lilium candidum (MADONNA LILY)
Perennial bulb to 1.5m with lance-shaped green foliage and fragrant, trumpet-like, white flowers in midsummer.

Treats skin ailments – ulcers, burns, bruises. Anti-epileptic properties.

Lythrum salicaria (PURPLE LOOSESTRIFE)
Perennial to 1 x 0.6m with lance-shaped, mid-green foliage and rose-red flowers in late summer.

General tonic. Antibiotic – for external wounds and eczema. Treats diarrhoea. Staunches bleeding. Eases menstrual problems.

LEFT Sunflowers add late summer colour to the garden and are commonly used in the treatment of throat or respiratory disorders.

Helianthus annuus (SUNFLOWER)
Annual to 3 x 0.3m with large, toothed, heart-shaped leaves and huge bright yellow flowers in late summer; edible and highly nutritious seeds. Many varieties available.

For all throat problems, asthma, coughs, colds. Brings down fever. Eliminates toxins for gout, rheumatism, arthritis, inflammation of kidneys.

Also for arrogant, vain people or those suffering from low self-esteem.

Helleborus niger (CHRISTMAS ROSE) ✖
Evergreen perennial to 30 x 45cm with dark green, leathery leaves and white flowers in midwinter.

Protects against all illness. Promotes menstrual flow. Heart stimulant for the elderly.

Hypericum perforatum (ST JOHN'S WORT)
Perennial to 90 x 90cm with pale green foliage and bright yellow, scented flowers in summer.

Antibacterial, antibiotic, antiviral properties – used in AIDS research. Sedative; soothes the nervous system and

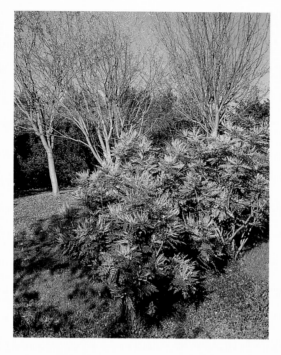

Mahonia aquifolium (OREGON GRAPE) ★
Evergreen shrub to 2 x 2m with leathery foliage;
scented yellow flowers in early spring followed by
blue berries.
General tonic for lethargy and during convalescence:
improves digestion, enhances appetite. Treats liver and
gall bladder problems. Detoxifier for rheumatism, arthritis,
gout. Eases skin conditions, including eczema and
psoriasis. Relieves problems with menstruation.
Enhances the immune system – inhibits tumour
development.
Also for people who are critical and dissatisfied or suffer
from paranoia.

Menyanthes trifoliata (BOG BEAN/BUCKBEAN)
Perennial aquatic to 25cm with mid-green, three-
parted leaves and racemes of pinky-white flowers in
early summer.
Tonic to relieve indigestion. Sedative. Eases menstrual
and rheumatic pain.

Monarda didyma (BERGAMOT)
Perennial to 90 x 60cm with aromatic, hairy, mint-
like foliage and whorls of sage-like, scarlet flowers
all summer; other varieties available.

Induces sleep. Eases colds, sore throats and catarrh.
Relieves nausea and menstrual pain.

Myosotis sylvatica (FORGET-ME-NOT)
Biennial to 40 x 30cm with small, oval, hairy leaves
and pale blue flowers in spring.
Relieves respiratory problems.
Also enhances relationships and eases feelings
associated with loss.

Myrtus communis (MYRTLE)
Evergreen shrub to 3 x 2.5m with dark green,
aromatic, leathery leaves, scented white flowers in
late summer and purple-black berries.
Antiseptic and astringent – heals wounds, psoriasis,
bruises. Relieves disorders of the respiratory, digestive
and urinary systems.
Lifts the spirits, especially in children.

Nepeta cataria (CATNIP/CATMINT)
Aromatic herbaceous perennial to 1 x 0.6m with
downy, nettle-like foliage and whorls of white or
lavender flowers in midsummer.
Relieves respiratory infections, decongestant for
bronchitis and colds. Relieves fever. Stimulates the
circulation. Good for rheumatism and arthritis. Relaxant,
including to digestive tract (for colic). Eases period pain,
normalizes periods. Relieves headaches and tension.
Energizes those with digestive or metabolic imbalances.

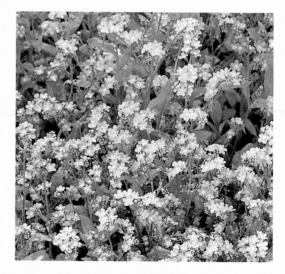

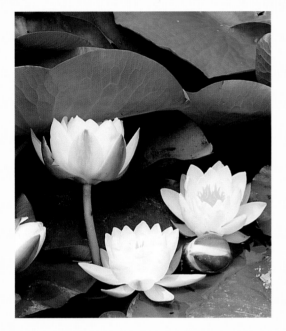

Nymphaea alba/N. odorata (WATER LILY)
Perennial aquatic with large, floating, round leaves
and large, white, fragrant flowers in summer. Other
varieties available.
Used for gynaecological problems, including infection.
Calming and sedative – for irritable bowel syndrome.
Relieves catarrh. Eases pain in kidneys and lower back.
Also for shyness or inhibition, and as an aphrodisiac.

Oenothera biennis (EVENING PRIMROSE)
Biennial to 1.5 x 0.45m with long green leaves and
clear yellow, cup-shaped, fragrant flowers through
summer.
Contains gamma-linoleic acid for healthy immune,
nervous and hormonal systems. Soothes skin problems,
including eczema, acne, allergies. Sedative. Relieves
digestive disorders, including diarrhoea and cramps.
Antispasmodic – for asthma. Good for circulatory
problems, including high blood pressure, high cholesterol
levels, blood clotting, coronary artery disease, heart
flutters. Eases metabolic problems, including multiple
sclerosis. Treats pre-menstrual syndrome and
menopausal problems. Counteracts alcohol damage
to liver.
Also for those who feel rejected and lack emotional
support.

Papaver somniferum (OPIUM POPPY) ✖
Annual to 1 x 0.3m with silvery, lobed leaves and
flowers in a range of pinks, purple or white in
summer; double flowers available.
Narcotic properties – unripe seeds are the source of
opium. Relaxant, analgesic and aphrodisiac properties.

P. rhoeas (RED POPPY)
Annual to 60 x 30cm with hairy, divided leaves and
scarlet flowers with black blotch at base in summer.
Similar action to opium poppy but milder. Sedative,
relieves headaches. Relaxes the intestinal tract – for colic.
Relieves coughs, bronchitis and asthma and clears the
respiratory system.

Passiflora incarnata (PASSION FLOWER) ★
Semi-evergreen climber to 9m with lobed leaves,
unusual purple and white flowers in summer
followed by golden fruit.
Relaxant – cures insomnia, relieves stress and tension.
Analgesic for headaches, neuralgia, shingles. Improves
the circulation; lowers blood pressure. Antispasmodic –
eases Parkinson's disease, asthma.
Also helps find one's inner self.

Persicaria bistorta (BISTORT)
Perennial to 60 x 60cm with long, oval leaves and
spikes of pink or red flowers in late spring.
Relieves urinary and stomach problems, ulcers, irritable
bowel syndrome, diarrhoea. Staunches blood flow for
haemorrhoids. Eases sore throats and coughs, treats
catarrh.

Polemonium caeruleum (JACOB'S LADDER)
Perennial to 60 x 30cm with pinnate leaves and
clusters of cup-shaped, lavender-blue flowers from
late spring.
Reduces fever. Treats epilepsy, nervous disorders and
headaches.

Polygonatum x hybridum (SOLOMON'S SEAL)
Perennial to 1 x 0.45m with pale green, oval foliage
and clusters of dangling, whitish-green flowers in
late spring followed by black berries.

LEFT Although water
lilies need open water,
some of the less vigorous
cultivars can be grown
successfully in a large
barrel or similar container.

RIGHT The Pasque flower (*Pulsatilla* sp.) produces wonderfully silky foliage and seedheads; it makes a good tonic for the nerves and also relieves many problems relating to women's health.

Aids tissue repair. Eases menstrual problems. Tonic for the respiratory system.

Polypodium vulgare (POLYPODY)
Evergreen fern to 40 x 40cm with leathery, mid-green, pinnate fronds.
Treats constipation, indigestion, jaundice, hepatitis. Supports the respiratory system – bronchitis, catarrh and coughs.

Populus balsamifera (BALSAM POPLAR)
Deciduous tree to 30 x 10m with fragrant, heart-shaped, glossy foliage and yellow catkins in spring followed by fluffy white seeds.
General tonic. Antiseptic – relieves coughs and bronchitis. Eases stomach and kidney complaints, rheumatism.

Primula veris (COWSLIP) ★
Herbaceous perennial with rosettes of wrinkled leaves and scented yellow flowers to 15cm in spring.
Tonic for the nervous system; relaxing and sedative for migraines, tension headaches. Treats skin problems, including acne, wounds, allergies. Antirheumatic, soothes pain. Provides protection from strokes – prevents blood clotting. Antispasmodic action for asthma. Relieves coughs, bronchitis, colds and chills.
Lifts the spirits, eases depression. Improves the memory and strengthens brain function.

Prunella vulgaris (SELF HEAL)
Perennial to 50 x 30cm with pointed oval leaves and violet or pink flowers.
Staunches bleeding of all wounds, soothes insect bites. Reduces inflammation, including gout. Relieves headaches, high blood pressure. Reduces fever. Treats lymphatic problems.
Also enhances inner healing powers in those who are unwell or unhappy; reduces dependence in addicts.

Pulmonaria officinalis (LUNGWORT)
Herbaceous perennial to 30 x 30cm with green, hairy leaves spotted with white and pinky-blue flowers in spring.

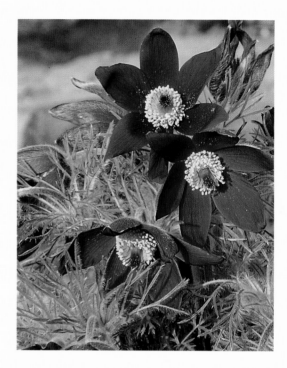

Relieves all chest conditions including bronchitis, wheezing, asthma, tuberculosis.

Pulsatilla vulgaris (PASQUE FLOWER) ★
Perennial to 25 x 25cm with silky grey foliage and purple bell-shaped flowers in spring.
Tonic for the nervous system – enables relaxation, eases emotional distress. Relieves fever. Analgesic. Good for disorders of the female reproductive system, including pre-menstrual syndrome, childbirth and post-natal depression.
Also enhances inner strength and improves the expression of emotions.

Rhus glabra (SMOOTH SUMACH)
Deciduous shrub to 5 x 5m with toothed, pinnate, blue-green foliage and spikes of hairy red flowers in summer, followed by fruits.
Eases diarrhoea. Relieves sore throats. Reduces fever. Diuretic. Useful in diabetes.

Ruta graveolens (RUE) ★ ✘
Evergreen shrub to 90 x 90cm with deeply divided, blue-green leaves and clusters of greenish-yellow flowers in early summer.

Regulates menstruation. Treats epilepsy, colic, eye problems and multiple sclerosis. Stimulates the appetite. Eases rheumatism, arthritis and neuralgia.

✖ Phototoxic: may provoke severe skin reaction after contact in sunlight.

Salix alba (WILLOW)

Deciduous tree to 20 x 10m with long green leaves and catkins in spring.

Provides aspirin – used to bring down fevers, treat rheumatic and arthritic problems, aches and pains, flu. Astringent – staunches bleeding. Reduces fluid retention and eliminates toxins. Improves the circulation (prevents blood clotting). Eases reproductive problems and menopausal symptoms (hot flushes and sweats).

Sambucus nigra (ELDER)

Deciduous tree or hedgerow shrub to 5 x 5m with dull green, pinnate foliage with an unpleasant smell; however, cream flowers in spring have a floral scent; edible purple-black fruits produced in late summer.

Relieves fever. Treats respiratory problems and infections, including coughs, colds, hay fever and catarrh; decongestant. Cleanses the system of toxins; relieves rheumatism, gout and arthritis. Sedative, relaxant – eases asthma. Mildly laxative.

Also imparts inner strength and allays fear during times of change.

Santolina chamaecyparissus (COTTON LAVENDER)

Evergreen shrub to 60 x 90cm with silvery-white, thread-like foliage and bright yellow flowers in summer.

Insect repellent. Regulates menstruation. Cleanses the kidneys.

Saponaria officinalis (SOAPWORT) ✖

Herbaceous perennial to 90 x 60cm with small, oval leaves and pink or white flowers in midsummer.

Expectorant; clears coughs, bronchitis and asthma. Eases rheumatic pain. Relieves skin conditions including eczema, acne and psoriasis.

Scutellaria lateriflora (SKULLCAP)

Perennial to 90 x 60cm with nettle-like foliage and small, pinky-blue flowers in summer.

Tonic for nervous system – for exhaustion, tension, headaches, depression, stress; useful during convalescence. Antispasmodic – calming for heart palpitations, epilepsy and cramps. Treats pre-menstrual syndrome and menopausal problems. Anti-inflammatory and reduces fever – eases arthritis, rheumatism and neuralgia. Stimulates the liver, used for urinary conditions. Aids withdrawal from drugs.

Silybum marianum (MILK THISTLE)

Biennial to 1.2 x 0.6m with glossy, spiny, dark green leaves marbled with white; purple-pink, thistle-like flowers in summer.

Stimulates the appetite. Relieves travel sickness. Treats cardiovascular disorders.

Stachys officinalis (BETONY)

Perennial to 60 x 30cm with dark green, aromatic, toothed leaves and spikes of pink-purple flowers in summer.

Nerve tonic and sedative – relieves headaches, tension, migraine, insomnia, panic attacks, shingles. Eases congestion. Purifies the blood. Improves digestion. Anti-spasmodic.

Symphytum officinale (COMFREY) ✖

Herbaceous perennial to 1 x 0.6m with large, hairy leaves and cream and pinkish-blue flowers in summer.

Skin problems – bruising, eczema, ulcers. Aids external healing of fractures or swellings. Anti-inflammatory action for arthritis, irritable bowel syndrome. Eases respiratory conditions including bronchitis.

✖ Phototoxic: avoid exposure to foliage during sunlight.

Tanacetum parthenium (FEVERFEW) ★

Perennial to 60 x 45cm with yellow-green, aromatic foliage and small, white, daisy-like flowers all summer; golden-leaved variety adds colour; double flowers also available.

Tonic to the nervous system. Mild sedative; treats

convulsions, headaches, migraine. Reduces pain and inflammation of rheumatoid arthritis. Reduces fever. Relieves menstrual problems. Used to treat asthma. Beneficial to the liver. Aids digestion, enhances appetite.

Taxus baccata (YEW) ✖

Evergreen tree to 12 x 7m with dark green, glossy, needle-like foliage and scarlet fruits on female plants.

Relieves rheumatic and urinary problems. Used in cancer treatment.

Thuja occidentalis (ARBOR VITAE) ★

Evergreen coniferous tree to 15 x 5m with scale-like, greeny-yellow leaves and small cones.

Relieves respiratory problems such as bronchitis. Diuretic – treats urinary infections, including cystitis. Eases stiffness in joints. Anti-viral – treats warts. Used in cancer treatment.

Tilia x europaea (LIME/LINDEN)

Deciduous tree to 30 x 15m with large heart-shaped leaves and pale yellow flowers with winged bracts in summer.

Relaxant and sedative – relieves tension and anxiety, depression, headaches and migraine, muscle tension, palpitations. Improves blood circulation, reduces high blood pressure, relieves arteriosclerosis and other heart problems, including congestion. Flushes toxins out of the body; reduces fever; treats colds.

Also heals emotional problems.

Trillium erectum (BIRTH ROOT) ★

Perennial to 45 x 30cm with whorls of three large, mid-green leaves and red-brown flowers in late spring.

Relieves menstrual problems of all kinds and eases childbirth. Staunches bleeding internally and externally, including ulcers. Antiseptic – heals skin problems, bites. Antispasmodic. Aphrodisiac.

Also of assistance to those who need material security and think possessions are the answer to their problems.

Tropaeolum majus (NASTURTIUM)

Trailing annual to 1.5m with rounded foliage and edible red, orange or yellow flowers through summer. Useful companion plant.

General tonic; enhances the immune system. Cleanses the system and relieves infection, particularly in the urinary tract (such as cystitis) or of the chest; clears catarrh, eases bronchitis. Increases circulation. Improves digestion; stimulates the liver and bowels.

Also for those who are drained by mental activity – balances intellectual and spiritual bodies.

Valeriana officinalis (VALERIAN)

Perennial to 1 x 1m with dark green, narrow leaves and pink or white scented flowers through summer

BELOW Said to ease childbirth, *Trillium erectum* produces unusual whorls of three leaves and bell-shaped flowers. It only thrives in true woodland conditions.

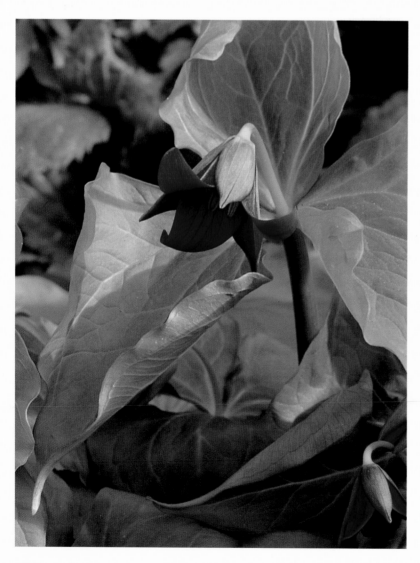

and autumn; variegated and golden-leaved forms also available.

Tonic for the nervous system – remedy for anxiety, stress, tension, headaches and epilepsy. Sedative; reduces blood pressure. Relaxant – eases colic, asthma, irritable bowel syndrome and spasm.

Verbascum thapsus (GREAT MULLEIN) ✖

Biennial to 2 x 0.6m with woolly, silver leaves and spires of yellow flowers through summer.

Diuretic with cooling properties – treats cystitis and aids the elimination of toxins to ease gout and arthritis. Treats respiratory problems such as coughs, asthma, whooping cough, bronchitis and tuberculosis. Cleanses the lymphatic system and clears congestion. Antiseptic and analgesic properties. Sedative – relieves tension and eases headaches, migraine and earache. Heals skin infections, eczema and wounds.

Also provides inner strength to deal with indecision.

Viburnum opulus (CRAMP BARK/GUELDER ROSE)

Deciduous shrub to 4 x 4m with lobed leaves and white flowers in spring followed by red fruit; golden-berried and dwarf forms available.

Eases all cramps and pains including swollen glands. Relaxes muscle tension – helps with asthma, period pain, colic, irritable bowel syndrome, nervous tension. Improves blood flow, reduces blood pressure.

Vinca minor (LESSER PERIWINKLE) ★

Evergreen trailing plant to 20 x 90cm with shiny, oval leaves and blue flowers in spring; other varieties available.

Astringent – stops bleeding of all types. Clears catarrh. Benefits the nervous system – reduces anxiety. Reduces blood pressure, treats arteriosclerosis. Relieves cramps and skin inflammation. Useful in diabetes.

Also useful for those prone to depression or nervous disorders including seasonal affective disorder (SAD).

Viola odorata (SWEET VIOLET)

Perennial to 15 x 40cm with dark green, oval leaves and sweetly scented purple or white flowers in spring.

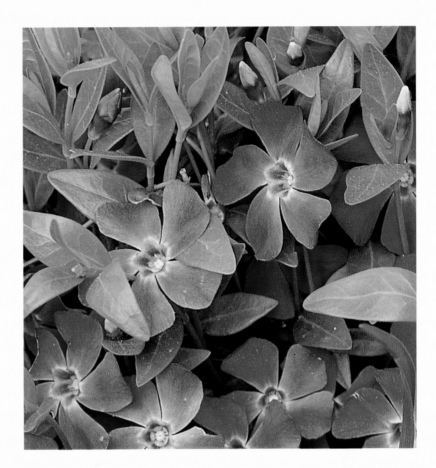

Nerve and heart tonic. Eases insomnia. Eliminates bladder and kidney stones. Soothes coughs, bronchitis, catarrh and chest infections. Reduces fever and inflammation (similar properties to aspirin) – headaches, rheumatism and arthritis. Cancer remedy.

Also supports the shy and timid and is said to heal the heart; the scent is conducive to meditation.

Viola tricolor (HEARTSEASE)

Annual to 30 x 30cm with dark green, oval leaves and purple, white and yellow pansy flowers throughout summer.

Treats heart complaints – strengthens the capillaries, reduces blood pressure and arteriosclerosis. Soothes the respiratory system – for coughs, asthma and bronchitis. Anti-inflammatory properties – for skin problems such as eczema and psoriasis, and for gout and arthritis. Reduces fever. Diuretic and blood-cleansing – relieves cystitis.

Also for the lonely, rejected and broken-hearted.

ABOVE Lesser periwinkle is available in many selected forms, including this one, *Vinca minor* 'Atropurpurea'. It may be useful in the treatment of a variety of conditions, including Seasonal Affective Disorder.

Bach flower remedies

Edward Bach was a renowned English physician who practised as a homeopath during the first half of the twentieth century. Trained in orthodox medicine, he held the holistic belief that true health depends on a harmony of body, mind and spirit and that all physical illness stems from negative thoughts or feelings. He saw that inner stresses depleted the immune system and lowered the body's natural resistance to disease. A negative mindset also appeared to hinder recovery. Dr Bach believed that if a balance could be found, the body would be healed.

Bach sought cures from nature for such imbalances, and found them mostly in the form of wild flowers, trees and herbs. He divided the most common negative states of mind into seven groups: fear, uncertainty, lack of interest in the present, loneliness, over-sensitivity, despair, and excessive concern for others. These are further divided to cover more specific feelings, for which he developed a system of thirty-eight remedies. The remedies are prescribed according to the patient's psychological state, not necessarily any physical complaint. The plants, he believed, could restore vitality so that those affected by disease could find the inner resources to bring about their own healing – in other words, it is the patient, not the disease, who needs treatment.

Dr Bach intended his remedies for self-help; they are sold in concentrated form and can be diluted in water, dropped on to the tongue, or rubbed on to the lips or behind the ears. Three or four remedies may be taken together. The Bach remedies act in a similar way to the 'vibrational' healing methods of homeopathy, the extracted essence bringing about healing at a very subtle level. In the same way that we might grow any plant in the garden for its healing abilities, so too may these flower remedies be included so that their life force might lift our spirits and enable us to heal ourselves. If you feel a particular description applies to your present state of mind, think about including the appropriate plant in your garden. Plant a tree where you can sit beneath it and be embraced by its powers, or simply grow the perennials in a border where they might cast their healing action over you.

Only thirty-seven remedies are listed here; the thirty-eighth is rock water, taken from any pure, natural spring which is open to fresh air and sunshine. It is useful for people who aspire to personal perfection and concentrate on the self, sticking rigidly to a self-imposed route through life.

Oversensitivity

Agrimonia eupatoria (AGRIMONY)
Perennial to 90 x 60cm with mid-green leaves and spikes of starry, yellow flowers through summer.
For worriers who hide their troubles behind a brave face and those who avoid confrontation, perhaps using alcohol or drugs to cope.

Centaurium umbellatum (CENTAURY)
Biennial to 25cm with a rosette of leaves and clusters of pink flowers in summer.
For sensitive people who are easily upset; for those who can't say 'no' and are exploited by others.

Ilex aquifolium (HOLLY)
Evergreen shrub to 7 x 5m with leathery, spiny, dark green leaves and small, fragrant, white flowers followed by red berries on female plants.
For overwhelming feelings of anger, suspicion, jealousy or envy; a desire for revenge.

Juglans regia (WALNUT)
Deciduous tree to 35 x 25m with large, aromatic, glossy, pinnate foliage and yellow-green catkins followed by nuts.
Those distracted by others from their own life aims; helps to ease the transition during times of change in life.

Loneliness

Calluna vulgaris (LING/HEATHER)
Evergreen shrub to 60 x 75cm with bright green, scale-like leaves and white, pink or purplish, bell-shaped flowers in midsummer to autumn.
For feelings of loneliness, a need for company and to talk, those obsessed with their own troubles.

Hottonia palustris (WATER VIOLET)
Perennial water plant with divided, light green foliage and lilac or whitish flowers in summer.
For the reserved and self-reliant who are lonely and keep themselves to themselves.

Impatiens glandulifera (IMPATIENS/HIMALAYAN BALSAM)
Annual to 1.5 x 0.6m with fleshy green foliage and deep purple to white flowers throughout summer followed by exploding seed capsules.
For those who are irritable and impatient, wanting everything done without delay.

Fear

Aesculus x carnea (RED CHESTNUT)
Deciduous tree to 15 x 15m with large, palmate foliage and candle-like clusters of rosy-pink flowers in late spring followed by 'conkers'.
Obsessive concern for others' safety and welfare, often overlooking own problems.

Helianthemum nummularium (ROCK ROSE)
Creeping perennial to 25 x 75cm with small green leaves and clusters of bright yellow flowers in summer.
Sudden feelings of terror, panic or hysteria, including nightmares; also used in emergencies.

Mimulus guttatus (MONKEY FLOWER)
Perennial to 60 x 45cm with oval, toothed leaves and yellow, snapdragon-like flowers with red spots in summer.
Phobias and fear of known things, shyness.

Populus tremula (ASPEN)
Deciduous tree to 15 x 10m with rounded, grey-green foliage and yellow catkins in spring followed by fluffy white seeds.
For fears of the unknown, apprehension for no known reason and nightmares; for sensitive people in need of inner strength.

Prunus cerasifera (CHERRY PLUM)
Deciduous tree to 10 x 10m with oval green leaves and small white flowers in early spring followed by plum-like fruits.
Fear of losing control, including insanity or senility; irrational or suicidal thoughts.

Uncertainty

Bromus ramosus (WILD OAT)
Evergreen perennial grass to 2 x 0.3m with mid-green, hairy leaves and sprays of grey-green flowers in summer.
For the ambitious who feel dissatisfied but lack direction; helps find a path through life.

Carpinus betulus (HORNBEAM) Deciduous tree to 25 x 20m with veined, dark green leaves and green catkins in spring followed by small winged nuts in autumn.
For lack of strength, both physically and mentally, and a feeling of being over-burdened by everyday pressures.

Ceratostigma willmottianum (PLUMBAGO/CERATO)
Deciduous shrub to 1 x 1.2m with hairy, oval leaves and rich blue flowers in late summer.
Indecision and doubting your own abilities or judgement; constant seeking of advice and confirmation from others.

Gentiana amarella (FELWORT)

Perennial to 50 x 45cm with lanceolate, green leaves and tubular, purple flowers in late summer.

Treats self-doubt and worry in those who are easily discouraged and prone to despondency.

Scleranthus annuus (SCLERANTHUS)

Low-growing annual with narrow green foliage and tiny white flowers in late summer.

Indecision and constant mind-changing, mood swings.

Ulex europaeus (GORSE)

Deciduous shrub to 2 x 1.5m with tiny, dark green foliage and fragrant, yellow flowers in spring and sporadically throughout the year.

For feelings of hopelessness and despair with no positive outlook, utter pessimism.

Lack of interest in the present

Aesculus hippocastanum (WHITE CHESTNUT)

Deciduous tree to 30 x 25m with large, dark green, palmate foliage and white, candle-like flowers in late spring followed by 'conkers'.

An obsessive or overactive mind causing an inability to relax or concentrate; persistent unwanted thoughts.

Aesculus hippocastanum (CHESTNUT BUD)

Buds from above.

Inability to learn from mistakes, repetition of the same error; encourages deeper self-observation.

Clematis vitalba (OLD MAN'S BEARD)

Deciduous climber to 20m with lance-shaped foliage and small, fragrant, white flowers in spring followed by fluffy seedheads.

For those who can't live in the present with a tendency to daydream, lacking concentration and living in hope of happier times.

Lonicera caprifolium (HONEYSUCKLE)

Deciduous climber to 6m with light green, oval leaves and yellowish-white flowers in summer, followed by poisonous orange berries.

For those who live in the past and look back too much to happier days, with an inability to focus on the present; people who can't move on after a loss.

Olea europaea (OLIVE)

Evergreen tree to 10 x 10m with narrow, grey-green foliage and tiny, fragrant, white flowers in late summer followed by edible fruits; grow in a conservatory or in a container to overwinter indoors.

For mental and physical exhaustion, causing weariness in life; brings peace to those who work too hard and don't relax enough.

Rosa canina (WILD ROSE)

Deciduous shrub to 3 x 3m with oval, toothed leaves and pinkish-white flowers in early summer followed by red hips.

Treats apathy, those with no interest in life and resigned to their circumstances.

Sinapsis arvensis (MUSTARD)

Annual to 60 x 45cm with large, lobed, green leaves and yellow flowers through summer.

Severe, unexplainable depression or despair, like a dark cloud coming from nowhere.

Despondency or despair

Castanea sativa (SWEET CHESTNUT)

Deciduous tree to 30 x 15m with glossy, toothed, dark green foliage and spikes of small yellowish flowers in summer followed by spiny-husked, edible nuts.

Complete hopelessness and despair in those who are exhausted and have reached the limit of their endurance.

Larix decidua (LARCH)

Deciduous conifer to 30 x 15m with light green, needle-like foliage and small cones in autumn after insignificant flowers.

For those who, although capable, lack self-confidence and fear failure, leading to despondency.

Malus sylvestris (CRAB APPLE)
Deciduous tree to 6 x 5m with oval, mid-green leaves and pinkish-white flowers in spring followed by golden yellow 'crabs'.
For those who feel they need to be cleansed – from self loathing, feelings of shame or physical ailments.

Ornithogalum umbellatum (STAR OF BETHLEHEM)
Perennial bulb to 30 x 20cm with narrow, grassy leaves and clusters of starry white flowers in late spring.
For great unhappiness following a shock or bad news, including loss.

Pinus sylvestris (SCOT'S PINE)
Evergreen conifer to 25 x 10m with reddish-brown bark, blue-green needles and brownish cones.
Self-reproach and guilt in those who feel they haven't done well enough and are always apologizing.

Quercus robur (OAK)
Deciduous tree to 25 x 25m with oval, lobed foliage and green-yellow male catkins in spring followed by acorns in autumn.
For those who are normally strong and battle courageously against adversity and illness; people who cannot let go or relax from work.

Salix alba subsp. *vitellina* (GOLDEN WILLOW)
Deciduous tree to 15 x 10m with orange-yellow shoots, lanceolate, mid-green foliage and yellow catkins in spring.
For bitterness or resentment about misfortune and a negative feeling that life is unfair.

Ulmus procera (ENGLISH ELM)
Deciduous tree to 35 x 15m with toothed, dark green foliage and inconspicuous flowers followed by winged fruits in autumn.

For those who work hard and feel overburdened by responsibility and inadequacy, causing depression.

Excessive concern for the welfare of others

Cichorium intybus (CHICORY)
Perennial to 1.5 x 60m with mid-green, arrow-shaped, hairy leaves and clear blue flowers in late summer.
For possessiveness and interference or over-concern for others; for those who are in constant need of attention and the insecure.

Fagus sylvatica (BEECH)
Deciduous tree to 25 x 25m with oval, wavy-edged leaves and small beech 'nuts' in autumn.
For perfectionists with an intolerance of others, the overly critical.

Verbena officinalis (VERVAIN)
Herbaceous perennial to 1 x 60m with hairy, lobed, dark green leaves and small, pale lilac flowers from midsummer.
For those with fixed ideas who preach to others and struggle constantly; the over-enthusiastic who can appear fanatical; those prone to nervous exhaustion.

Vitis vinifera (GRAPE VINE/VINE)
Deciduous climber to 15m with large, lobed leaves and insignificant flowers followed by green or black fruits.
Treats dominance and over-forcefulness; inflexible, arrogant people.

Rescue remedy
For use in emergencies, crisis or trauma; the rescue remedy comforts and calms.
Mixture of impatiens, clematis, rock rose, cherry plum and star of Bethlehem. Perhaps you could plant these five together somewhere in your garden so that you have a ready-made remedy for times when you have received an unpleasant shock.

Chinese herbal medicine

Traditional Chinese medicine has been practised since at least 2500 BC, and is still in widespread use in China today, alongside orthodox methods. Often at odds with Western beliefs about health, the fundamental concept is that a life force (energy) or *ch'i* animates every aspect of the universe and that its condition in a person will influence their state of health. The flow of *ch'i* around the body, through a network of channels known as meridians, is commonly balanced through such techniques as acupuncture, diet and herbal medicine.

In Chinese medicine, no cause of illness is sought as disease is felt to be an expression of disharmony; an imbalance between *yin* and *yang*, the two opposite but complementary principles, neither of which can exist without the other. Different parts of the body are deemed to be relatively *yin* or *yang* and certain symptoms may also be categorized as such. Excess *yin* may present as a feeling of cold, dampness or shivering; where *yang* predominates, a patient may be hot and feverish. Thus warming herbs, such as ginger, are used to treat conditions caused by excess cold, whereas salty 'water' herbs, such as Chinese figwort, are prescribed for fluid imbalances. Emotional characteristics may also be caused by an imbalance of the five elements; for example, excess 'wood' may lead to uncontrollable feelings of anger, and where 'water' is overly dominant a person may be unnecessarily fearful and anxious.

Good health depends upon the harmonious interaction between *yin* and *yang* and the five 'elements'. The following describes the function of the five elements in more detail:

Wood relates to sour herbs, which nourish *yin*; these refresh, aiding digestion and liver function: Chinese dogwood berries, hawthorn berries, rose hips, schisandra.

Fire applies to bitter herbs, which are *yin* and cooling and will drain systems, detoxify, fight infection and stimulate the digestive system: burdock, dandelion, peony, Chinese rhubarb.

Earth relates to sweet herbs which, being *yang*, warm and soothe, acting as a tonic and providing nourishment: ginseng, Chinese angelica (*dong quai*).

Metal herbs are spicy or pungent and *yang*; their heating, drying properties will improve circulation, stimulate energy and digestion, and relieve arthritic pain: cinnamon, ginger, peppers, cloves.

Water herbs are salty and *yin*, cooling and moistening to support the kidneys and maintain fluid balance: seaweeds, barley, Chinese figwort.

Chinese medicine has begun to gain credibility in the West, where it has been found to be successful in the treatment of disorders which have proved difficult to treat with conventional drugs. For instance, extreme cases of eczema have responded to herbal treatment where every other approach has failed.

Once a Chinese practitioner has diagnosed an imbalance, he or she will prescribe an often complex mixture of herbs. These are generally taken in the form of a strained liquid after boiling the constituents (bark, roots, fruit or flowers) in water; extracts or pre-manufactured mixtures are rarely used. The prescriptions are entirely geared to the individual and vary according to many contributory factors; it is therefore impossible to self-prescribe and home treatment should not be attempted.

However, using the principles of homeopathy (see page 91) it is possible that the presence of certain plants in the garden may be enough to stimulate the body's self-healing powers.

The Chinese classification of herbs is perhaps the broadest known to man; it uses 6,000 medicinal plants, many of which are considered to be ornamental plants in the West. The following 'Chinese' herbs can all be grown successfully in a temperate climate:

Ailanthus altissima (TREE OF HEAVEN)
Deciduous tree to 20 x 12m with large, pinnate leaves and small greenish-yellow flowers in summer followed by winged fruits.
Treats digestive disorders and certain heart conditions. Antispasmodic – eases asthma. Possible anti-cancer properties.

Arctium lappa (BURDOCK)
Biennial to 1.5 x 1m with large, green leaves and reddish-purple, thistle-like flowers in summer.
Assists recovery from infection. Detoxifying – for gout, arthritis, and skin problems. Muscle relaxant. Anti-tumour action.

Clerodendrum trichotomum (GLORY BOWER)
Deciduous shrub to 3 x 4m with large leaves, clusters of fragrant, white flowers in late summer, followed by blue berries set in red calyces.
Analgesic – for joint pain. Relieves eczema. Lowers blood pressure.

Codonopsis pilosula (CODONOPSIS)
Climbing perennial to 1.5m with oval leaves and pendulous green and purple flowers in summer.
Tones *ch'i* throughout the body; for general fatigue, digestive problems and respiratory problems, including asthma. Increases endurance to stress (reduces adrenaline levels). Raises red blood cell levels and reduces blood pressure.

Corydalis solida (CORYDALIS)
Tuberous perennial to 20 x 15cm with narrow leaves and pinkish-red flowers in spring.
Sedative – reduces stress. Relieves abdominal and period pain. Invigorates blood flow after an injury for rapid healing.

Dianthus superbus (FRINGED PINK)
Annual to 45 x 20cm with narrow, mid-green foliage and fragrant, fringed, pink, white or lilac flowers in midsummer.
Tonic for the nervous system. Treats conditions of the kidneys and urinary tract. Eases constipation. Relieves eczema.

Eucommia ulmoides (GUTTA PERCHA)
Deciduous tree to 15 x 9m with elliptical, glossy, dark green leaves and inconspicuous flowers in spring.
Improves circulation. Tonic for liver and kidneys. Relieves lower back pain and weakness.

Forsythia suspensa (WEEPING FORSYTHIA)
Deciduous shrub to 3 x 2.5m with mid-green foliage and bright yellow flowers in early spring.

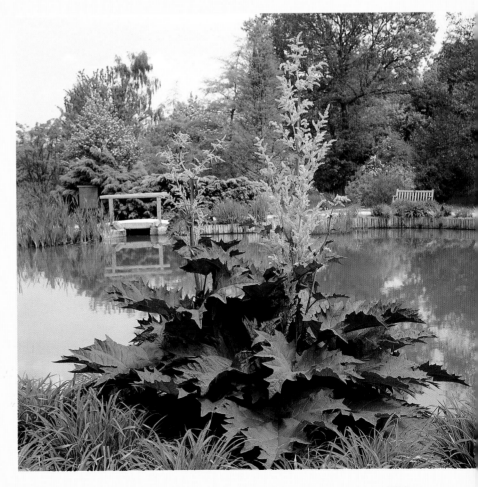

BELOW An ornamental form of rhubarb, *Rheum palmatum* is valued in Chinese medicine for its antibacterial properties. It is an attractive perennial plant which associates well with water and needs damp soil to thrive.

Antiseptic. Eases colds, flu and fever.
Used in treatments for breast cancer.

Ginkgo biloba (GINKGO) Deciduous conifer to 25 x 10m with unusual fan-shaped, bright green leaves, which turn yellow before they fall; female plants have foul-smelling fruit.
Improves circulation, particularly to the brain – aids memory, concentration and senile dementia. Anti-inflammatory; relieves coughs, wheeziness and asthma. Reduces risk of stroke and associated diseases.

Hemerocallis fulva (DAY LILY)
Perennial to 90 x 75cm with sword-like, light green leaves and orange flowers through early summer.
General tonic. Antibacterial properties. Some parts of the plant are poisonous.

Lonicera japonica (HONEYSUCKLE)
Semi-evergreen climber to 7m with oval leaves and fragrant, yellow-white flowers in summer followed by black berries.
Fights infections such as sores, inflammation and dysentery. Brings down fever.

Magnolia officinalis (HUO PO)
Deciduous tree to 15 x 10m with aromatic bark, large green leaves and fragrant cream flowers in spring.
Pain relief. Problems of the digestive tract, including indigestion.

Morus alba (WHITE MULBERRY)
Deciduous tree to 15 x 15m with rounded, glossy, deep green leaves and inconspicuous flowers followed by edible, whitish fruits in summer.
Expectorant – relieves catarrh. Reduces fever. Relieves dizziness, headaches and insomnia. Combats fluid retention. Eases joint pain. Treatment of diabetes.

Paeonia lactiflora (CHINESE PEONY)
Perennial to 1.5 x 0.9m with divided dark green leaves and large, silky-white, scented flowers.
Antibacterial and antiviral – heals cold sores. Reduces

fever. Antispasmodic, anticonvulsive, calming – treats headaches, nightmares, hysteria, fright, epilepsy. Helps menstrual disorders, menopausal symptoms. Lowers blood pressure. Remedy for kidney and gallstones and liver complaints. Treats congestion of the blood – wounds, poor circulation, varicose veins. Used during and after childbirth – but not during pregnancy, Some parts of the plant are poisonous.

Phyllostachys nigra (BLACK BAMBOO)
Evergreen shrub to 7m with clumps of brown-black stems and long, narrow mid-green leaves.
Detoxifier, diuretic. Brings down fevers.

Platycodon grandiflorus (BALLOON FLOWER)
Perennial to 60 x 45cm with blue-green, toothed foliage and clear blue or purple, bell-shaped flowers in summer.
General tonic. Cough remedy.

Prunus mume (JAPANESE APRICOT)
Deciduous tree to 10 x 7m with oval, bright green leaves and pinkish-white flowers in early spring followed by yellow fruit.
Antibiotic – eases coughs. Stops bleeding and diarrhoea. Treats corns and warts.

Rheum palmatum (CHINESE RHUBARB)
Perennial to 2 x 1.5m with large, lobed leaves and panicles of small, creamy-white or crimson flowers in early summer.
Treats constipation. Antibiotic.

Schisandra chinensis (MAGNOLIA VINE)
Deciduous climber to 8m with large, toothed leaves and pale pink flowers in late spring followed by red berries.
Stimulates nervous system – improves mental clarity, treats depression, prevents forgetfulness, Helps body adapt to stress and aids sleep. Eases respiratory problems and coughs. Balances fluid levels within the body. Protects and improves liver function (hepatitis). Treats skin rashes, including eczema. Sexual stimulant; stimulates contractions of uterus,

RIGHT The Chinese peony is available in many selected colours and double forms although the true type is stunning in its simplicity. In Chinese medicine, it is considered to have many useful properties and is a particularly valuable 'all-rounder'.

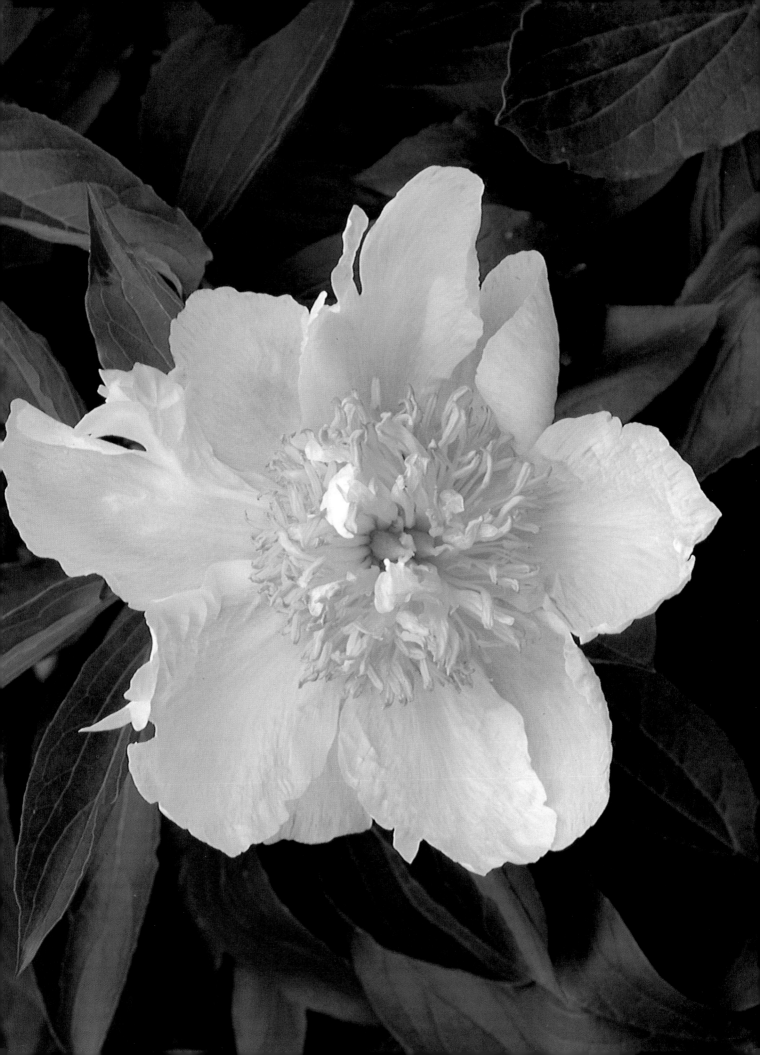

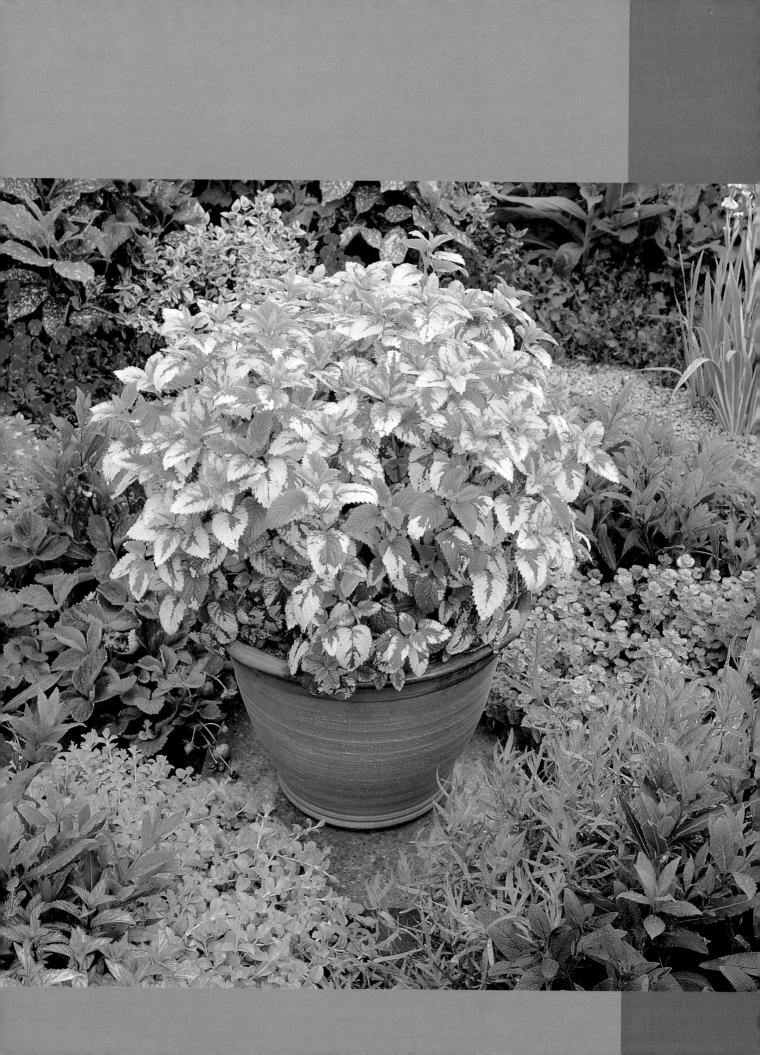

5 Aromatherapy

And because the Breath of Flowers is far Sweeter in the Air (where it comes and goes, like the Warbling of Musick), than in the Hand, therefore nothing is more fit for that delight, than to know what be the Flowers and Plants, that do best perfume the Air.

FRANCIS BACON

Aromatherapy is a relatively modern name for an ancient holistic practice. Practitioners use essential oils, extracted from a vast range of aromatic plants, to improve both physical health and mental well-being. Although the basis of this therapy was laid down thousands of years ago, the principles remain highly relevant today. It works through a combination of psychological action and molecular interaction. Both aspects have now been scientifically proven, but – although not expressed in quite the same terms – both were known to the ancients. The movement of scent molecules through the body via the circulatory system was noted by the Greek philosopher-physician Theophrastus, who demonstrated that an aromatic poultice applied to the leg could scent the breath. Aromatherapy is now one of the most widely practised complementary therapies and is currently used to treat a myriad of ailments, from rheumatism and migraine to stress. Why is it so popular? Apart from the proven potency of many plant essences, aromatherapy gives us something that is sometimes lacking in other alternative practices: quite simply, it has the power to make us feel good. Whether accompanied by a massage or simply used to scent the air around us, aromatherapy is an intensely enjoyable experience.

The phenomenal success of aromatherapy is such that it is not easy to buy any cosmetic product these days that does not claim to offer 'relaxing' or 'revitalizing' benefits. For many people, this approach conjures up images of potpourri, bubble baths and scented massage oils, yet these are simply elements of this multi-faceted practice. Just as we have seen in the previous chapter how herbs can be used to create a healing environment in our gardens, so too can an equally diverse range of fragrant plants, chosen specifically for their precious essential oils. Through careful selection of suitable species, our garden borders can be composed to refresh, relax, soothe or stimulate as required.

The aim of this chapter is to explain the principles of aromatherapy and to adapt the knowledge of the treatment room for use in our own gardens so that the benefits of the essential oils may be harnessed *in situ*. For the price of a single aromatherapy consultation, a small collection of plants can be bought to create an attractive corner of the garden with the potential to provide years of health benefits.

LEFT Variegated lemon balm (*Melissa officinalis* 'Variegata') makes an attractive centrepiece in this area. As with many golden forms, it is best grown in light shade so that the leaves do not scorch. In general, however, most plants grown for their fragrance do best in full sun, where the production of essential oils will be at its strongest.

Historical background

Widespread evidence suggests that men and women have always used fragrant plants to heal body, mind and spirit. Much of our present-day knowledge is based upon the use of essential oils in Egypt some 5,000 years ago. The ancient Egyptians are generally regarded as the founders of aromatherapy and they used the therapeutic powers of scented oils in everyday life. The essences, obtained from plants by a crude distillation process, were used medicinally, in perfumes and beautifying potions, for massages, as fumigants, in religious ceremonies (as mood-altering incense) and for embalming.

Perfumed plants were used regularly in ancient Greece, where many philosophers, including the physician Hippocrates, advocated a daily aromatic bath and massage to soothe away stresses and strains and prolong life. The practice was later taken up in Rome, the luxury of exotic fragrance sitting well with the Romans' sensual lifestyle.

Meanwhile, throughout the Orient, the use of aromatics for health also thrived and the ancient civilizations of China, India and Arabia all made use of the fragrant plants at their disposal. Written evidence dating back to before 2000 BC demonstrates that the Chinese have harnessed the healing properties of certain plants over thousands of years, while the Ayurvedic medicine of India has used scented oils since at least 1000 BC. In the Middle East, the Persian physician Avicenna is credited with the invention of distillation in the eleventh century; this allowed the production of sophisticated aromatic oils and floral waters, which were used by Arab physicians for therapeutic massage and to scent the air and fight disease.

From the twelfth century onwards, knights returning from the Crusades brought knowledge of perfumery and distillation back to Europe, and for many centuries this knowledge was used in conjunction with herbalism to prevent and cure all manner of ills. During the Great Plague of 1665, Londoners burnt bundles of aromatic herbs in the streets and carried sweet-smelling posies as a defence against infectious disease.

However, as synthetic drugs have been developed to fight disease, the popularity of herbal medicine has waned throughout the Western world. A few interested parties continued their research but, for the most part, the use of medicinal plants has been sadly neglected.

The aromatherapy we know today was developed by a French chemist, René-Maurice Gattefossé, in the 1920s. Gattefossé discovered that extracts distilled from certain aromatic plants had a profound effect on the body; like many great discoveries it began with an accident, when he burned his hand in his laboratory. He treated the burn with lavender oil and found that the wound healed remarkably quickly. He published many books, including *Aromatherapy*, which described the therapeutic properties of essential oils. The book was read by Jean Valnet, a French army doctor who began his own research and, during World War II, successfully used essential oils to treat soldiers suffering from both battle wounds and psychiatric disorders.

In the 1920s, two Italian doctors were able to demonstrate that the sense of smell has a psychotherapeutic influence over the function of the central nervous system.

In the 1950s, biochemist Marguerite Maury studied the effectiveness of oils when absorbed through the skin. She developed the methods used in aromatherapy today, of diluting essential oils, blending them in individual recipes and applying them through massage.

Robert Tisserand was one of the first authors in English on the subject. *The Art of Aromatherapy*, published in 1977, has done much to initiate interest in the subject worldwide.

Modern aromatherapy

Aromatherapy has truly come of age since the 1980s. Today, biochemists continue to investigate the properties and benefits of essential oils. They have now isolated dozens of active ingredients that account for some of the incredible properties of healing plant essences. In many instances, folklore can now be substantiated by scientific fact.

Many European aromatherapists are also doctors, since it is illegal in some countries to present oneself as a 'therapist' without a medical qualification. The study of essential oils is included in many medical schools, and in countries such as Germany and Switzerland the benefits of essential oils are so widely accepted that it is even possible to recoup the cost of treatment through health insurance. The therapy has been shown to be particularly good at relieving stress-related problems; anxiety, depression and insomnia; muscular and rheumatic pains; digestive disorders; menstrual and menopausal complaints. Unlike allopathic treatments, aromatherapy works with the body, rather than against symptoms, and, with a few exceptions, side effects are rare.

Essential oils are very concentrated and although a tiny bottle of oil may seem expensive, a little goes a long way. The essential oil should never be applied directly to the skin. Scent molecules enter the body through inhalation and/or absorption through the skin, using techniques such as:

- Massage – essential oils must be diluted in a carrier oil, in order to avoid skin reactions and aid absorbency. Preferably use a cold-pressed oil such as almond, hazelnut or grapeseed (not baby or cooking oil), and mix approximately six drops of essential oil (two or three different ones) with 2 teaspoons (10 ml) of carrier oil.
- Bathing – add a few drops of two or three different oils (six to eight drops in total, or half that quantity if you are pregnant) to a warm (not hot) filled bath and agitate the water before you get in. It won't leave a greasy 'tide mark' because the oil molecules are so tiny. The oil can be diluted in a carrier or bath oil, particularly if you have dry skin. Relax for quarter of an hour.
- Inhalation – add three or four drops of oil(s) to a large bowl of hot water, mix well and cover your head with a towel; inhale the vapour for a few minutes, keeping your eyes closed. Alternatively the oils can be applied to a handkerchief and sniffed occasionally, taking care to avoid direct contact with the skin.

These treatments are particularly good for treating colds and coughs, and clearing the head. Inhalation is not recommended for asthmatics.
- Vaporization – essential oils can be used in a variety of burners to create a certain mood in a room (or even on a still summer's night in the garden). Always follow the instructions for your particular burner and take care near a naked flame as essential oils are highly flammable. Alternatively a room can be scented by a few drops of essential oil on a piece of cotton wool behind a radiator.

If you have a particular health problem, rather than a more general need for relaxation or revitalization, the choice of essential oils can be bewildering, and it might be a good idea to consult a qualified aromatherapist. They will ask questions about your health and general lifestyle before suggesting appropriate oils.

Some of the essential oils commonly used by aromatherapists are derived from plants that grow only in tropical climates. Since this book is intended primarily for gardeners in temperate climates, oils such as ylang ylang, sandalwood and patchouli will not be considered in this chapter.

Because aromatherapy works at a molecular level, it is possible to assume that growing plants for their aromatic properties is likely to have similar benefits to treatments using essential oils. Furthermore, this interpretation of aromatherapy should, under normal circumstances, lead to no dangerous side effects. If the plants are not consumed nor any parts applied directly to the skin, there is very little chance of harm, even for those in certain 'risk groups', such as pregnant women (however, see page 131).

Finally, an important point to bear in mind is that the botanical names used in aromatherapy are often trade terms and are not always the names of the species from which the oil derives. Many of the essential oils used, for instance lavender, come from plants which have been bred and grown purely for medicinal purposes. The varieties commonly found in our gardens will often be less productive in terms of their oils than commercial species.

The power of scent

There is, perhaps, nothing more evocative than scent. Our sense of smell is so finely tuned that most people can identify more than 10,000 different aromas and this range can often be enhanced through training. It is also remarkably personal; to some, a scent might appear strong and musky, while others perceive it to be light and floral.

It remains a mystery why some people can only detect certain scents or perceive fragments of others. The answer may lie partly in the individual power of smell, partly in our ability to describe what the scent is truly like. We might attempt, in the manner of wine tasters, to attach descriptions to aromas such as 'heavy' or 'fruity', but much of the vital essence simply does not translate into words. Instead we tend to compare one fragrance with another and find it extremely hard to describe a fragrance to someone who has never smelt it for themselves.

Scent can have a magical quality, often conjuring up distant and personal memories. Once experienced, scents are rarely, if ever, forgotten and are able to stir deep emotions within us; we can be powerfully affected by the fragrances in our everyday lives. This is because our sense of smell is closely linked with our memory and we often recollect people, places or events in connection with certain aromas from our pasts – our mother's perfume, father's pipe smoke, grandparents' kitchen...

When we inhale an aroma, scent molecules are taken into the lungs, stimulating sensory cells in the upper nasal passage (olfactory tract) as they pass. The molecules diffuse across the lining of the lungs into blood capillaries and thence into the blood-stream, which circulates them around the body. The molecules travel to various systems or organs where they exert their therapeutic effect; scientists have found that certain scent molecules will always gather in specific parts of the body, thus they can be linked to specific ailments. Although brought about relatively quickly, the health benefits can last for many hours after initial exposure to the scents.

As we inhale them, these same molecules are detected, through nerve impulses, by the olfactory area of the brain. This lies within the limbic system, in the brain's right hemisphere. This zone is concerned primarily with emotion, intuition, memory and creativity; smell is the only sense that has a direct link to this part of the brain. This explains the particularly powerful memories we tend to associate with scent. Once an aroma is detected, it is categorized and the hypothalamus and pituitary bodies are stimulated to produce an appropriate response to the mood provoked by the particular smell. These reactions go on to affect the autonomic nervous system and hormonal system, which govern heart rate, digestion, and feelings of anger, fear and stress. A number of biochemical responses then occur throughout the entire body. This chain of events supports the concept of holistic health, where every action, thought and emotion is linked.

The new science of psychoneuroimmunology demonstrates that an unhappy mental state can theoretically lower our resistance to all manner of physical ills. These may initially be very minor, such as colds, but they have the potential to become much more serious with time. The flip side of the coin, however, is that pleasurable experiences – that create a happy state of mind – can have healing powers. A generally happy and positive outlook can strengthen our natural immunity.

Aromatherapy should therefore be an enjoyable experience; if an aroma is perceived as pleasant, endorphins (happiness chemicals) are released to create a feeling of well-being. Using EEG instruments to record the electrical activity of brain and skin, research is now being carried out into the response of the central nervous system to specific aromas. Scientists have discovered that 'sweet' essences such as mimosa or chamomile produce alpha, theta and delta brainwave patterns, implying a state of relaxation or even sleep. Other fragrances, such as rosemary, induce beta brainwaves; these are more

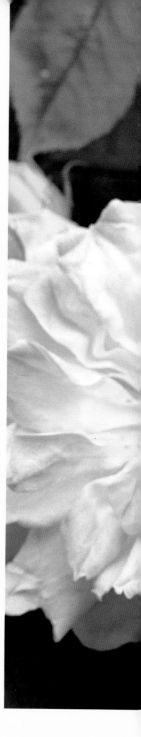

ABOVE Some roses are far more fragrant than others. When selecting a particular variety for aromatherapy, check the strength of its scent before you are bowled over by its colour and individual beauty.

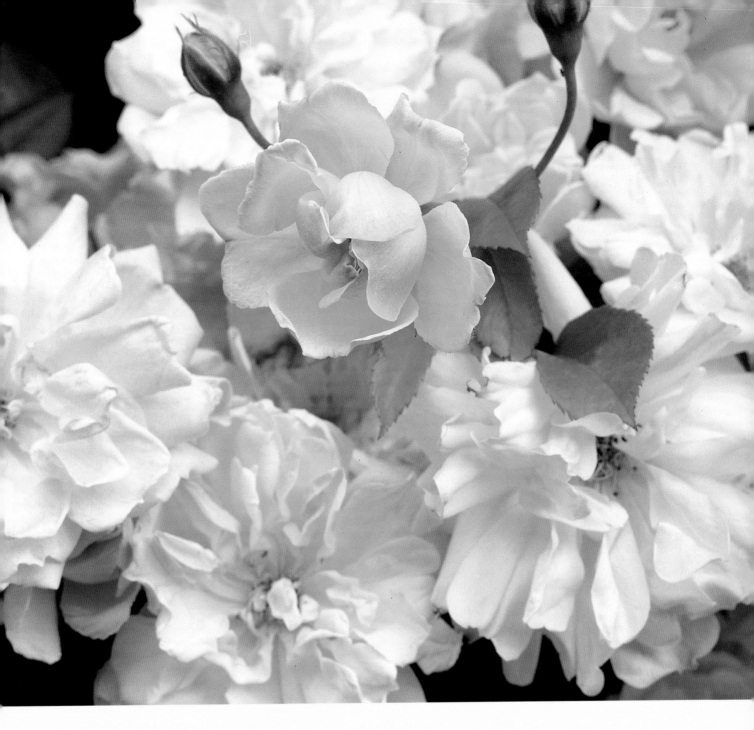

rapid patterns and denote a state of alertness. A few oils, for instance lavender and geranium, have a balancing effect; they either invigorate or sedate according to the needs of the individual. Interestingly, it appears that these reactions do not occur if an aroma is disliked; this appears to block any effect upon the nervous system. Perceptions of 'pleasant' and 'unpleasant' are, of course, highly subjective and past memories of a scent will affect an individual's reaction. This might help to explain why two people respond so differently to the same essence(s).

Research also demonstrates that people respond to fragrances so dilute that they can't actually smell them. It is believed that this response may be even more profound because the subconscious overrules the conscious mind so that we cannot fight the body's natural reaction. This discovery supports the fundamental belief of homeopathy and the Bach flower remedies (see page 116) – that a reaction is brought about even where the essence is so dilute that only the energy pattern, vibration or 'memory' of the original material remains. It is possible, therefore, that certain plants in the garden, growing in their natural state, have an active and relevant healing role. Such plants are, theoretically, capable of inducing a beneficial reaction simply through the release of minute quantities of essential oils through their leaves, flowers or fruit.

Essential oils

Essential oils (or essences) are considered by some to be the life force or 'soul' of a plant and by others to be possibly the DNA or plant hormones. Essential oils give fragrance to plants and are used to attract pollinating insects, repel predators and protect against disease. They are carried in the oil glands found in one or more parts of aromatic plants: the petals, leaves, seeds, fruits, roots, bark and stalks of different species are utilized and each has an individual characteristic. For example, the orange tree produces three entirely separate essences with varying medicinal properties: neroli (flowers), petitgrain (leaves) and orange (rind).

The chemistry of essential oils is incredibly complex: most consist of dozens of organic compounds such as terpenes, esters, alcohols and phenols. It is not simply the aroma of the oil but the whole plant essence which brings about the health benefits, since so many other molecular components are inhaled at the same time; a single oil can therefore often help a variety of disorders. For instance, lavender acts as an antiseptic and is also antibacterial, antibiotic, antidepressant, analgesic, decongestant and sedative. In fact, all essential oils have been found to possess antibacterial properties and many are also antifungal. Some, such as rosemary and juniper, are even antirheumatic; they stimulate the blood flow and lymphatic circulation, increasing the supply of oxygen to affected areas and aiding the elimination of the waste products which cause pain.

The essential oils used in aromatherapy (usually obtained by steam distillation) are highly concentrated liquids and, unlike ordinary vegetable oils, they tend to be volatile and will evaporate in open air. The quantity and quality of oil produced by a plant is determined by many factors and, just like a fine wine, alters from year to year, depending on climatic and other variations. Oil production will also be affected by soil type and fertility, the age of the plant and time of harvest. This last is important since oil concentration in flowering plants is generally highest at midday during warm, dry weather but this varies by species; jasmine is best harvested at night, damask rose immediately after the morning dew. Many oils are extremely expensive to produce because of the amount of plant material required; for example some 60,000 rose flowers are required to make one single drop of the essential oil.

Aromatherapy for specific problems

The practice of aromatherapy uses pure essential oils for the treatment of a myriad of ailments. When grown in the garden, plants may have a more subtle effect than if the extracted essential oil were used, but as described earlier, even in minute quantities the benefits can be measured.

The science of psychoneuroimmunology (see previous page) has shown that smelling pleasant fragrances can, by balancing the mind/body equilibrium, help to strengthen the body's immune system. This in turn will improve the body's defences against the dangers of viruses, allergens, environmental pollution and stress. Aromatherapy can help stress by 'nipping it in the bud', combating its build-up at source before symptoms change from relatively minor problems into major illness.

Bearing in mind the holistic approach, the powers of aromatherapy are arguably at their strongest when used to prevent the onset of illness rather than simply relieve the symptoms. For this reason, long-term problems, such as low immunity, arthritis, chronic depression, and certain illnesses, for example hepatitis and Parkinson's disease, require full medical attention. A qualified aromatherapist should be consulted before attempting any home treatment.

In addition to physical complaints, aromatherapy also effectively treats psychological problems or imbalance. It can improve our mental state, helping us to cope better with grief, depression or mental fatigue. The following can all be planted in the garden for their general beneficial effects:

Stimulating	Balancing	Relaxing	Anti-depressant
ANGELICA	BASIL	CEDARWOOD	BASIL
CARNATION	GERANIUM	CHAMOMILE	CARNATION
CITRUS	LAVENDER	CLARY SAGE	CHAMOMILE
EUCALYPTUS	ROSE	CYPRESS	CITRUS
FENNEL	VALERIAN	HOPS	CLARY SAGE
JASMINE	VIOLET LEAF	JUNIPER	GERANIUM
PEPPERMINT	YARROW	MARJORAM	JASMINE
PINE		MELISSA	LAVENDER
ROSEMARY		MIMOSA	ROSE

During pregnancy, many essential oils are prohibited (*see below*). The following, however, are particularly recommended, but only after the first trimester: CITRUS, CYPRESS, GERANIUM, LAVENDER, PINE, ROSE.

Side effects

All extracted essential oils should be treated with respect, since they are powerful substances; a few are even toxic in undiluted form. The isolation of the 'active principles' of plants has created some highly effective remedies and potentially dangerous drugs such as atropine (deadly nightshade). These synthesized drugs can cause severe side effects which are, however, extremely rare with 'whole' plant treatments. This is because the numerous trace chemicals within each essential oil not only increase efficacy, but also buffer the potentially harmful side effects of any individual ingredient. Unmodified oils, as released naturally by plants in the garden, are even safer to use due to this natural synergy.

Another important consideration is that essential oils are far less likely to have harmful side effects if they have been harvested from plants grown under organic conditions. For this reason (and many equally relevant ones) plants should be grown without the use of chemical fertilizers or sprays.

There are, however, some people who are potentially more likely to be affected by allergic reactions. If you suffer from hay fever, asthma, eczema, food allergies, or have a particularly sensitive skin, you may also have a sensitivity to one or more essences and should exercise more caution than most. The following essences are most likely to trigger allergic reactions in sensitive people: BASIL, CARNATION, CEDARWOOD, CHAMOMILE, CLARY SAGE, FENNEL, GRAPEFRUIT, HOPS, JUNIPER, LAUREL/BAY, LEMON, MELISSA, ORANGE, PEPPERMINT, PINE, THYME. None, if simply brushed past in the garden, should cause problems.

In addition, sufferers of epilepsy should avoid the following essences: FENNEL, ROSEMARY.

The following essences are photosensitizing; exposure to sunlight should be avoided after contact since they may cause skin blistering: ANGELICA ROOT, CITRUS (FROM THE FRUIT PEEL).

Many women find that their sense of smell and preferences alter during pregnancy, so planting might need to be adjusted in the short term. In addition, pregnant women should take great care with certain plants; the following should be avoided during pregnancy: ANGELICA, BASIL, CEDARWOOD, CHAMOMILE, CLARY SAGE, FENNEL, JASMINE, JUNIPER, LAUREL/BAY, MARJORAM, PEPPERMINT, ROSEMARY, TARRAGON, THYME, YARROW.

The aromatherapeutic garden

Can there be any better way to enjoy the therapeutic effects of plants than directly as nature intended? Everyone can include scented plants within their garden and, with a little planning, the healing powers of aromatherapy may be harnessed through the selection of appropriate species. Since the chemical composition of essential oils alters as soon as the material is harvested, it makes sense to take advantage of the plants when they are at their most potent, that is when they are still alive and growing.

A qualified aromatherapist might use between thirty and eighty essential oils. However, not only would it be impossible to grow this range of plants in the average garden, it would also be counterproductive to blend more than three or four in any one area. Initial selection will be governed by the practical constraints of a particular garden – its location, climate, space and soil type – as well as by cost, personal preference and availability. Nevertheless, there will always be at least one plant to satisfy both practical requirements and the more esoteric ones of its owner. The selection of plants should be carried out by those who intend to use the area for its health benefits. It is vital to act on your own feelings and use the plants which smell 'right' to you. Whatever choices are made, bear in mind the need to orchestrate a pleasing combination of plants (see page 142).

Many of the individual plants offer a myriad of benefits and if space is restricted, it pays to select the most versatile species. Equally, there is often some choice when it comes to plants which exert the same beneficial influence. For instance, if your aim is to create an area to relieve stress, and you only have a tiny town garden at your disposal, clary sage, geranium and rosemary may be used in place of large trees such as pine. In the smallest garden, a simple rose-covered bower will aid relaxation and soothe a headache. For those with the most minuscule gardens, even a group of pots or a window box can play host to a useful selection of scented plants. If you have more available land, a mixture of juniper, eucalyptus and pine might be planted in order to ease general aches and pains.

Generally, plants – especially herbs such as rosemary, basil, and thyme – will produce more essential oils when grown in full sun, and the release of volatile oils will be highest on a hot day. Others, such as violets, valerian and angelica, prefer to grow in a little shade and tend, on the whole, to be less highly scented. Try to choose plants that suit the times you most use the garden. If you only sit out during balmy summer evenings, select those which release their strongest fragrance at dusk, for example jasmine, night-scented stock (*Matthiola bicornis*) or tobacco plants (*Nicotiana* spp.).

In order to make the most of the perfume released, it is best to plant in a sheltered area so that the aromas do not dissipate too quickly on a breeze. Also bear in mind the height of the plant. Low-growing species such as carnations and chamomile are best grown in pots or raised beds so that their scent can be enjoyed without having to bend down to ground level. Place fragrant winter flowers close to a path so that you don't have to struggle through muddy ground on a freezing day just for a whiff of mahonia or witch hazel.

To ensure the most potent oil production from the plants in our gardens we need to encourage healthy growth, applying appropriate nutrients to stimulate leaves, flowers or fruit as required. Organic nitrogen fertilizers will encourage lush, leafy vegetation in non-flowering subjects such as eucalyptus, spruce and juniper, while high potash fertilizers will assist flowering and fruiting in subjects such as rose, lemon, fennel and hops.

Aromatic plants for a healing garden

AILMENT/CONDITION	ANGELICA	BASIL	BIRCH	CARNATION	CEDAR	CEDARWOOD	CHAMOMILE	CLARY SAGE	CYPRESS	EUCALYPTUS	FENNEL	GERANIUM	GRAPEFRUIT	HOPS	JASMINE	JUNIPER	LAUREL/BAY	LAVENDER	LEMON	MARJORAM	MELISSA	MIMOSA	ORANGE	PEPPERMINT	PINE	ROSE	ROSEMARY	SPRUCE	TARRAGON	THYME	VALERIAN	VIOLET	YARROW
ALLERGIES *see chapter 2*																																	
Asthma		◆					◆	◆	◆	◆				◆				◆	◆	◆	◆			◆	◆	◆	◆			◆			
Hay fever							◆			◆								◆			◆				◆	◆							
CIRCULATION																																	
High blood pressure							◆	◆										◆	◆	◆					◆								◆
Low blood pressure						◆			◆	◆		◆								◆				◆	◆		◆			◆			
Circulatory problems		◆	◆			◆	◆	◆	◆			◆				◆	◆	◆	◆					◆	◆	◆	◆	◆		◆		◆	◆
RESPIRATION																																	
Colds and flu	◆	◆				◆			◆	◆						◆	◆	◆	◆					◆	◆	◆	◆	◆		◆		◆	
Congestion	◆	◆				◆			◆	◆				◆	◆			◆	◆	◆	◆			◆	◆	◆	◆	◆		◆			
PAINFUL JOINTS																																	
Arthritis and rheumatism	◆		◆		◆	◆	◆		◆	◆						◆	◆	◆	◆	◆				◆	◆		◆	◆		◆		◆	◆
Muscular aches and pains	◆	◆				◆	◆		◆	◆		◆			◆	◆	◆	◆	◆	◆				◆		◆	◆	◆		◆			
STRESS RELATED																																	
Exhaustion	◆	◆					◆		◆	◆	◆				◆	◆	◆	◆						◆	◆	◆		◆		◆			
Anxiety		◆			◆	◆	◆	◆	◆			◆		◆	◆	◆		◆	◆	◆					◆		◆			◆	◆	◆	
Headache/migraine	◆	◆					◆	◆				◆						◆		◆				◆		◆	◆			◆		◆	
Insomnia		◆					◆	◆						◆	◆	◆		◆		◆	◆				◆						◆		◆
Mild depression		◆		◆			◆					◆	◆		◆	◆		◆	◆		◆	◆	◆	◆	◆	◆				◆			
Mental fatigue	◆	◆							◆	◆		◆	◆					◆	◆					◆	◆	◆	◆			◆	◆		
Frayed nerves							◆	◆						◆				◆	◆	◆			◆		◆						◆		◆
To strengthen the nerves							◆									◆		◆															
Normalizing/balancing *(lifts or soothes as needed)*		◆										◆						◆						◆		◆				◆	◆	◆	◆
Grief															◆			◆		◆				◆									
Digestive disorders	◆						◆				◆							◆	◆	◆	◆		◆	◆					◆	◆			
PRE-MENSTRUAL SYNDROME	◆		◆		◆	◆	◆	◆	◆		◆	◆			◆	◆	◆	◆		◆	◆				◆				◆				◆
AVOID DURING PREGNANCY	◆	◆	◆			◆	◆	◆			◆				◆	◆	◆			◆				◆					◆	◆	◆		◆

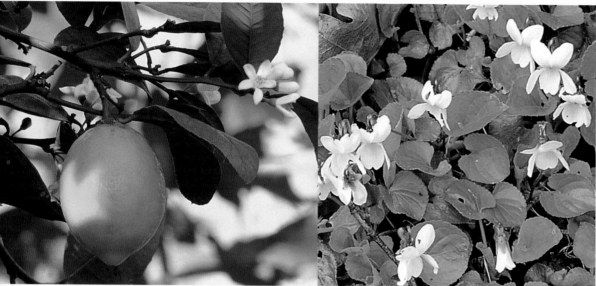

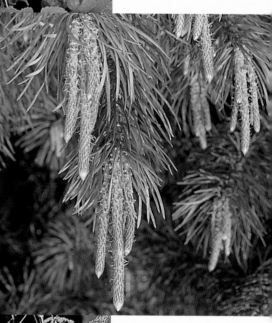

Five fragrance families

CLOCKWISE FROM TOP LEFT You might need a conservatory to enjoy the fragrance of the 'citrus' family such as this lemon; the sweet scent of violet (here *Viola odorata* 'Alba') typifies the 'florals'; pine needles are used to produce a 'green' fragrance; fennel seeds exude a 'spicy' aroma and are the source of its essential oil; the fragrance of cedar (here *Cedrus atlantica* 'Glauca') is described as 'woody' or balsamic.

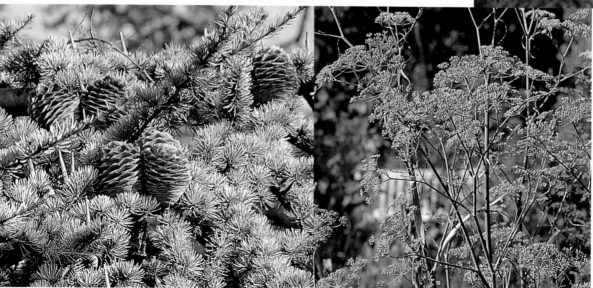

Fragrance families

Essential oils are grouped according to their general effects and fall into one of five fragrance families: green, citrus, floral, spicy or woody. The following pages feature temperate species only, although some may require winter protection. Certain warnings are sometimes given to those undergoing aromatherapy with essential oils. These should be borne in mind, although side effects will be minimal when plants are growing in the garden.

✖ Avoid contact in sunlight

★ Do not use if pregnant

Not to be used by people with epilepsy

♥ Not to be used by young children

◆ Allergy sufferers should avoid exposure to plant

Citrus

Citrus	Healing uses	Scent associates well with
GRAPEFRUIT ✖◆ Peel (*Citrus paradisi*) Small evergreen tree with dark green glossy leaves and wonderfully fragrant white flowers followed by large yellow fruits. Best grown in a conservatory or container as it requires winter protection.	General tonic or pick-me-up Refreshing, uplifting Muscle fatigue Nervous exhaustion	LAVENDER EUCALYPTUS JUNIPER GERANIUM CITRUS CYPRESS PINE ROSEMARY
LEMON ✖◆ Peel (*Citrus limonum/limon*) Small evergreen tree, producing strongly scented pinky-white flowers followed by bright yellow fruits. Best grown in a conservatory or container as it requires winter protection.	Eases cold symptoms and asthma, clears the head General digestive problems Improves blood circulation Insect repellant Skin problems	ROSE EUCALYPTUS CITRUS JUNIPER LAVENDER CYPRESS CHAMOMILE MARJORAM
ORANGE ✖◆ Peel (*Citrus sinensis*) Evergreen tree, producing clusters of fragrant white flowers followed by fruit; the flowers and fruit are often found on the plant at the same time. Best grown in a conservatory or container as it requires winter protection.	Relaxant, eases aches and pains Detoxifies the liver Aids sluggish digestive systems Refreshes and stimulates the over-tired or stressed	ROSEMARY CLARY SAGE GERANIUM LAVENDER CITRUS

Floral	Healing uses	Scent associates well with
CARNATION ◆ Flowers (*Dianthus caryophyllus*) Low-growing perennial, approximately 45 x 45cm with bluish-green foliage and clusters of small pinky-purple flowers borne on long stems in midsummer.	Antidepressant Antifungal properties	CEDARWOOD CITRUS CLARY SAGE LAVENDER
GERANIUM Leaves, flowers (*Pelargonium graveolens*) Spreading shrub growing to a height of 1m with rose-pink flowers; the entire plant is aromatic. This plant will require winter protection from frost.	Soothes problem skin Relaxant for anxiety, tension, stress Relieves menstrual problems Mood enhancer, balancing effect Insect repellant	JASMINE CITRUS LAVENDER ROSEMARY CLARY SAGE CYPRESS CEDAR CHAMOMILE JUNIPER
JASMINE ★◆ Flowers (*Jasminum officinale*) Vigorous evergreen climber growing to 9m, producing masses of fragrant, white, star-shaped flowers throughout summer. The powerful fragrance intensifies after dusk.	Alleviates grief, stress, fatigue Eases symptoms of pre-menstrual syndrome and menopause, including irritability Uplifting, relaxing, sensual Soothes muscular aches and pains	FLORALS CLARY SAGE CITRUS
LAVENDER Flowering tops (*Lavandula officinalis/angustifolia*) Evergreen shrub growing to 1 x 1m with grey-green leaves and bluish-mauve flowers in dense spikes at the end of wiry stems through summer.	Stress headaches Insomnia Encourages skin healing Eases painful joints and sprains Relieves high blood pressure Balances nervous system Digestive problems Period pains, pre-menstrual syndrome Insect repellant	CLARY SAGE JUNIPER GERANIUM PINE CEDARWOOD CITRUS ROSE MARJORAM EUCALYPTUS CHAMOMILE CYPRESS
MIMOSA Flowers, twig ends (*Acacia dealbata*) Evergreen tree with attractive silver-green ferny leaves and fragrant, yellow, fluffy flowers borne in long sprays during spring. Best grown in a conservatory or container as it requires winter protection.	Pre-menstrual syndrome General pick-me-up to cheer the spirits and treat depression Soothes nervous tension	LAVENDER CEDARWOOD ROSE GERANIUM

Floral (continued)	Healing uses	Scent associates well with
ROSE Petals (*Rosa damascena/R. centifolia*) Deciduous shrubs growing to 1.5 x 1.2m with prickly stems and large fragrant flowers in summer. *Rosa centifolia* bears globular pale pink flowers; *Rosa damascena* has deep pink double flowers.	Headaches Stress-related conditions, insomnia and depression Mood enhancer, uplifting Pre-menstrual syndrome and menopause Allays grief	CEDARWOOD CHAMOMILE CITRUS FLORALS CLARY SAGE
VIOLET Leaves, flowers (*Viola odorata*) Small herbaceous perennial, growing to 15 x 40cm with fragrant violet or white flowers in spring.	Boosts the circulation, thus easing rheumatism Improves concentration and clears the head, relieves headaches Eases emotional turmoil	ANGELICA FLORALS YARROW

Green

	Healing uses	Scent associates well with
BASIL (French) ★◆ Leaves, flowering tops (*Ocimum basilicum*) Tender culinary herb with highly aromatic glossy leaves and white flowers; grows to 60 x 30cm, best cultivated in pots. The variety 'Dark Opal' bears dark metallic-purple leaves.	Calming yet uplifting Useful for insomnia, anxiety, stress Soothes muscular aches and pains Regulates the menstrual cycle Improves circulation, respiration	CYPRESS EUCALYPTUS GERANIUM ROSEMARY LAVENDER LEMON CLARY SAGE JUNIPER PEPPERMINT
CHAMOMILE (Roman) ★◆ Flowers, leaves (*Chamaemelum nobile*) Low-growing herb to 25 x 40cm with finely cut feathery evergreen leaves and small daisy-like white flowers on single stems in summer.	Relaxant, relieves anxiety and nervous tension Digestive disorders Skin irritation and allergies Period pains, menopausal problems Sedative – treats insomnia and relieves stress Headaches Anti-allergic properties for asthma	LAVENDER GERANIUM CLARY SAGE JASMINE CITRUS ROSE
CLARY SAGE ★◆ Flowering tops (*Salvia sclarea*) Strongly aromatic, hardy annual herb growing to 75 x 90cm with spikes of white, blue, violet or pink flowers (bracts) in midsummer.	Relaxes and soothes headaches, sedative effect Strengthens the nervous system and relieves stress and depression Lowers blood pressure Eases menstrual problems Infertility	MIMOSA JUNIPER JASMINE PINE LAVENDER ROSEMARY

Green (continued)	Healing uses	Scent associates well with
EUCALYPTUS ♥ Leaves and twigs (*Eucalyptus globulus*) Tall evergreen tree growing to 30m and requiring protection in colder areas. The mature leaves are blue-green and sickle-shaped with clusters of cream flowers in spring.	Powerful antiseptic Stimulating, improves circulation Decongestant – clears the head and assists breathing Soothes muscular aches and pains Useful for skin problems Insect repellant	CEDARWOOD THYME ROSEMARY LAVENDER MARJORAM LEMON PINE GRAPEFRUIT PEPPERMINT
MARJORAM ★ Leaves, flowers (*Origanum vulgare/marjorana*) Perennial herb growing to 30 x 30cm with rounded greyish leaves and small white or purplish flowers arranged in clusters during midsummer. The variety 'Aureum' has young yellow leaves which fade to green.	Warming, eases aches and pains including rheumatism Soothes digestive problems, anxiety, insomnia Headaches Relieves period pains Calms and relaxes when tired or stressed	LEMON LAVENDER EUCALYPTUS ROSEMARY GERANIUM JUNIPER BAY CHAMOMILE
MELISSA ◆ Leaves, flowering tops (*Melissa officinalis*) Perennial herb growing to 60 x 45cm with bright green aromatic leaves and small white flowers in summer. The variety 'All Gold' has golden foliage.	Allergies including asthma, eczema Insomnia, migraine and anxiety Relieves high blood pressure Eases menstrual problems Nervous exhaustion and stress Digestive problems	CITRUS CHAMOMILE LAVENDER GERANIUM ROSE
PEPPERMINT ★ ♥ ◆ Leaves, flowers (*Mentha piperita*) Invasive perennial herb growing to 60 x 60cm with mid-green leaves on reddish stems and lilac flowers in summer.	Soothes muscular pain Decongestant Eases mental fatigue, headaches, migraine Soothes digestive problems, relieves nausea, indigestion and flatulence Insect repellant	EUCALYPTUS LAVENDER LEMON CLARY SAGE GERANIUM JUNIPER
PINE ◆ Needles, twigs (*Pinus sylvestris*) Evergreen coniferous tree growing eventually to 30m. The mature bark is orangish and needles are a bluish grey-green.	Useful for viral infections Soothes aching muscles and arthritis Invigorating, improves circulation Relieves fatigue and stress Insect repellant	CYPRESS BIRCH CEDARWOOD EUCALYPTUS LAVENDER JUNIPER LEMON ROSEMARY

Green (continued)	Healing uses	Scent associates well with
ROSEMARY ★ # Flowering tops (*Rosmarinus officinalis*) Evergreen flowering shrub growing to 1.8 x 1.8m. The leaves are leathery and very narrow with white felt beneath. The bluish, two-lipped flowers in late spring resemble tiny orchids.	Invigorating pick-me-up or tonic Refreshes nasal passages and assists breathing Relieves headaches Eases arthritis and rheumatism Improves circulation Soothes aches and pains	PEPPERMINT CEDARWOOD LAVENDER CITRUS, BASIL THYME PINE, BAY
SPRUCE/EASTERN HEMLOCK Needles, twigs (*Tsuga canadensis*) Evergreen coniferous tree growing eventually to 30m, bearing dense, dark green, yew-like foliage and solitary cones.	Reduces anxiety and stress Boosts circulation Soothes aching limbs and rheumatism Eases congestion of coughs and colds	BASIL CHAMOMILE EUCALYPTUS JUNIPER LEMON THYME ROSEMARY
THYME ★ ◆ Leaves, flowering tops (*Thymus vulgaris*) Hardy perennial growing to 20 x 30cm with small evergreen leaves and tiny mauve flowers arranged in clusters at the tops of upright stems. The variety 'Aureus' has golden variegated leaves.	Powerfully antiseptic and antiviral Treats nervous tension, headaches, fatigue – acts as stimulant Soothes rheumatic aches and pains Eases breathing problems Aids digestion Insect repellant	MARJORAM BIRCH CHAMOMILE ROSEMARY LAVENDER LEMON CLARY SAGE SPRUCE

Spicy

CYPRESS Needles, twigs and cones (*Cupressus sempervirens*) Narrow evergreen coniferous tree growing to 15m in warmer areas. The aromatic grey-green foliage is held in erect sprays and the cones are glossy and grey-brown.	General tonic – boosts circulation, eases rheumatism Soothes menstrual or menopausal problems Calms and relieves tension, stress Improves breathing – colds, asthma	CITRUS JUNIPER GERANIUM CLARY SAGE BIRCH LAVENDER PINE, BAY
FENNEL ★ # ♥◆ Seeds (*Foeniculum vulgare*) Short-lived perennial growing to around 2m x 45cm with feathery green leaves and flat heads of small yellow flowers in summer. The variety 'Purpureum' has bronze foliage.	Treats indigestion and flatulence Loss of appetite, nausea Pick-me-up for those suffering from exhaustion Menopausal problems, pre-menstrual syndrome and fluid retention	BIRCH CEDARWOOD ROSE GERANIUM VALERIAN LAVENDER CHAMOMILE ROSEMARY

Spicy (continued)	Healing uses	Scent associates well with
Hops ◆ Female flowers (*Humulus lupulus*) Herbaceous climber growing to 6m (with support) with lobed green leaves and clusters of flowers in summer. The variety 'Aureus' has golden foliage.	Eases breathing – asthma Relieves headaches, insomnia Relieves nervous tension and stress Menstrual and menopausal problems	Cypress Juniper Lavender Pine
Juniper ★◆ Berries (*Juniperus communis*) Small evergreen coniferous tree of variable habit. It has bluish-green prickly needles and produces an abundance of blue-black berries which are used to flavour gin. The variety 'Stricta' forms a narrow columnar tree to 3.5m.	Cleanses the system – hangovers Relieves tired muscles, aching limbs, improves circulation Treats water retention, menstrual problems including pre-menstrual syndrome Relieves stress	Rosemary Lemon Lavender Geranium Birch Cypress
Laurel/Bay ★◆ Leaves (*Laurus nobilis*) Evergreen shrub growing eventually to 9m – can be clipped to keep it in check. Dark leathery leaves and insignificant flowers followed by black fruits on female plants.	Boosts immune system Soothes aches, pains and rheumatism Relieves pre-menstrual syndrome, especially cramps	Cypress Eucalyptus Juniper Lemon Pine Birch Cedarwood Rosemary Lavender
Tarragon ★ Leaves (*Artemisia dracunculus*) Aromatic perennial herb growing to 1m with narrow green leaves and small heads of greenish flowers in summer.	Eases stomach complaints and flatulence Treats pre-menstrual syndrome and cramps, reduces water retention Soothes rheumatic pain	Basil Birch

Woody/balsamic

Angelica ✖ ★ Seed, roots (*Angelica archangelica, A. officinalis*) Tall biennial herb growing to 2m with attractive bright green ferny leaves and umbels of whitish-green flowers in summer.	Relieves menstrual problems Eases muscular aches and rheumatism Soothes indigestion, flatulence, colic Speeds the healing of cuts or bruises Useful for migraine, stress, fatigue	Clary sage Violet Geranium Citrus Rose Chamomile Eucalyptus Lavender Mimosa

Woody/balsamic (continued)	Healing uses	Scent associates well with
BIRCH (white) Leaf buds, bark (*Betula alba, B. pendula*) Graceful deciduous tree growing to 20m with white, peeling bark and diamond-shaped green leaves. Catkins are produced in early spring.	Soothes skin problems, eczema Antifungal Prevents water retention Improves circulation – relieves rheumatism	BAY CYPRESS FENNEL JUNIPER GERANIUM LEMON PINE TARRAGON THYME
CEDAR ★ Wood (*Cedrus atlantica*) Evergreen coniferous tree growing eventually to around 30m. Silvery-green leaves are arranged in tufts and long cones are produced.	Useful for stress-related conditions General stimulating tonic Eases arthritis, rheumatism Relieves pre-menstrual syndrome	BAY FLORALS ROSEMARY ORANGE CLARY SAGE CYPRESS JUNIPER
CEDARWOOD ★◆ Wood (*Juniperus virginiana*) Evergreen coniferous tree growing to 6 x 1.8m. Dark green needle-like leaves on slender branchlets.	Harmonizing tonic, relieves stress Stimulates tired, aching muscles Eases symptoms of catarrh Menstrual problems including pre-menstrual syndrome	GERANIUM ROSEMARY ORANGE CLARY SAGE ROSE CYPRESS JUNIPER JASMINE EUCALYPTUS
VALERIAN Roots (*Valeriana officinalis*) Herbaceous perennial growing to 1 x 1m with deeply cut leaves and clusters of white, pink or mauve flowers in summer.	Eases nervous tension Powerful sedative effect, overcomes insomnia Acts as mood enhancer	CHAMOMILE FENNEL GERANIUM LAVENDER ORANGE
YARROW ★ Leaves, flowers (*Achillea millefolium*) Herbaceous perennial growing to 75 x 60cm with aromatic, dark green, ferny foliage and flat heads of white flowers in early to midsummer.	Eases menstrual problems Calms the nerves, lowers blood pressure Sedative – eases insomnia and stress Improves circulation – for arthritis	CHAMOMILE GERANIUM JUNIPER ORANGE ROSE VIOLET LAVENDER CLARY SAGE

Planting mixes

One of the great pleasures of aromatherapy in the garden is the huge range of possibilities that exist for creating personalized blends through plant associations. Whatever your preferences, needs or environment, an appropriate mix of plants can be selected. When starting to think about the effect you are hoping to achieve, it is important to make your choices in a positive frame of mind as this will affect your final selection.

Beyond the constraints of influences such as climate and soil type, the most important factor at the outset is that all of the plants you believe to be suitable have scents which you find agreeable. If you choose aromas that you dislike, perhaps because you know the plant will grow well in your neighbourhood, the healing effect will be lost. Your reaction to a particular scent has a profound effect upon the outcome of exposure to that plant and it is vital that you are comfortable with the feelings and emotions it suggests. Interestingly, aromatherapists report that many people find they are instinctively drawn to the plant essence(s) suiting their physical or emotional needs at a particular time; it is quite common to go off certain aromas when their healing properties are no longer required. Therefore, always be led by your instincts and intuitive response.

A combination of blended essences often has a more powerful healing effect than ingredients used singly. This demonstrates the principle of synergy, that the effect of the whole is greater than the sum of the parts. On the other hand, mixing more than three or four essences tends to be counterproductive and the beneficial actions will be lessened. When grouping plants together, the ideal is to create a balanced, harmonious, mood-enhancing mixture where no one fragrance overpowers the others. Take care when combining strongly scented plants with those of subtle fragrance, but remember that the numbers can be adjusted to increase or lessen the effect of a particular species. Some 'heavier' scented plants, such as honeysuckle, jasmine and lilies, should be included with restraint as many people find them overpowering, particularly in the evening. As a guide, the following are listed in descending order of fragrance intensity:

Very high – CARNATION, MIMOSA, VALERIAN
High – ANGELICA, BASIL, CHAMOMILE, EUCALYPTUS, FENNEL, HOPS, JASMINE, MELISSA, PEPPERMINT, ROSE, THYME, YARROW
Fairly high – CLARY SAGE, GERANIUM, MARJORAM, ROSEMARY
Medium – JUNIPER, LAVENDER, CITRUS, PINE, ROSE
Low – CEDARWOOD

Bear in mind that in general, essences within the same fragrance family blend well together, for instance 'florals' such as geranium with rose and 'greens' such as chamomile with clary sage. 'Citrus' scents also blend well with both 'spicy' and 'woody' fragrances. Some essences – for instance eucalyptus, peppermint, fennel, thyme and chamomile – can be overwhelming and care should be exercised when growing them alongside other plants, especially florals. Appropriate blends are suggested alongside each plant within its fragrance family on pages 135–141, but these are by no means exhaustive; experiment to find the mix that suits you best.

Another principle to bear in mind is that used by the perfume industry, which defines three separate types of aroma: 'top', 'middle' and 'base' notes. In most commercial scented products, these three notes are combined to create a fragrance that is fuller and longer lasting than any individual scent. The blended layers are detected at different times to extend the overall appeal of the perfume.

The top note is detected first and is ephemeral, being the quickest to disperse. This scent adds lightness, it is often smelt from a distance, and it awakens and stimulates the senses, then disappears to reveal the middle note. Examples are basil, citrus, eucalyptus, laurel/bay, peppermint, tarragon, thyme (also mock orange blossom, wisteria, sage and alyssum).

Middle notes impart fullness to the fragrance, being neither too light nor too heavy, and smell the same close up as from a short distance away. Examples are carnation, chamomile, clary sage, fennel, geranium, jasmine, juniper, lavender, marjoram, melissa, mimosa, pine, rose, rosemary (also lily-of-the-valley and bluebells).

Base notes are resinous, earthy or woody and have a profound influence on the whole blend. In perfumery they act as a fixative to improve the scent's staying power and they linger long after the other notes have faded. The are generally soothing and calming. Examples are cedarwood, cypress, angelica (also lilac).

It is worth noting that some plants have the ability to release different scents throughout the day, for example jasmine, honeysuckle, mock orange blossom and mignonette.

BELOW This small bed contains a host of aromatic plants. Besides rose and clary sage (whose essential oils are used in aromatherapy) are tobacco plants (*Nicotiana*), purple sage (*Salvia officinalis* 'Purpurascens') and mock orange (*Philadelphus coronarius* 'Aureus').

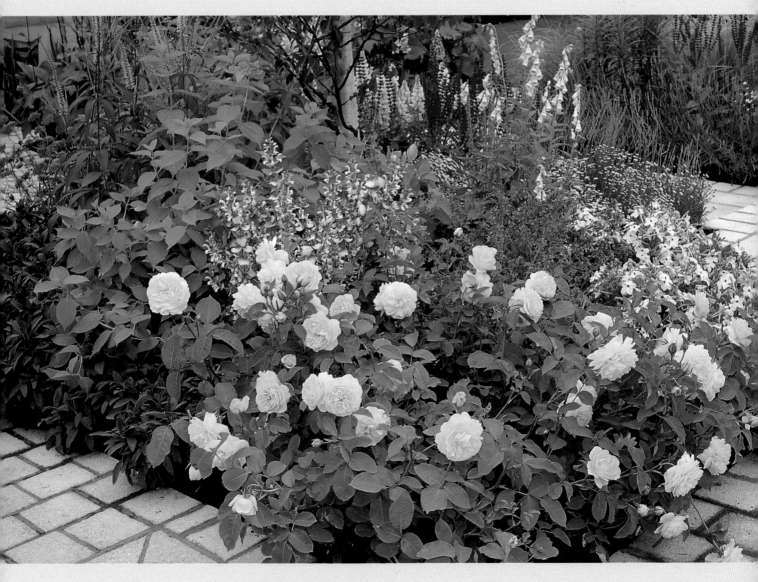

Widening your horizons

Unscented plants can be included in the aromatherapeutic garden to complement the fragrant varieties and enhance a particular mood. Think about their colours: blues, mauves, whites, creams and soft yellows will have a calming effect, while the warmer tones of red, orange and stronger yellows will enliven and revitalize body, mind and soul.

In addition to the plants listed on pages 135–141, many fragrant plants which are not used in true aromatherapy may be useful where they complement the overall effect you are trying to achieve. The following list, which is by no means exhaustive, may be helpful. Many are ideally suited to small spaces such as a terrace or windowsill; those marked thus ★ are particularly useful.

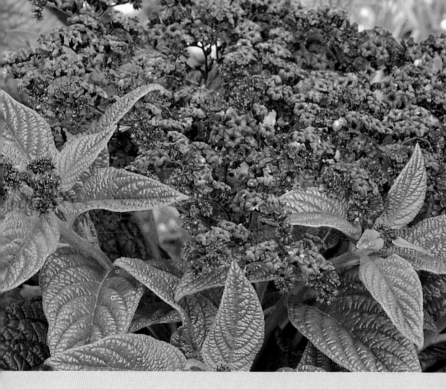

BELOW The rich purple flowers of the annual heliotrope emit a powerfully sweet scent which is often described as similar to 'cherry pies'.

Spring

Berberis x stenophylla (BARBERRY)
Buddleja globosa (ORANGE BALL TREE)
Convallaria majalis (LILY-OF-THE-VALLEY)
Daphne odora 'Aureomarginata'
Erysimum cheiri (WALLFLOWER) ★
Fraxinus ornus (FLOWERING ASH)
Hyacinthoides non-scripta (BLUEBELL)
Hyacinthus orientalis CVS. (HYACINTH) ★
Iberis saxatalis (CANDYTUFT) ★
Magnolia stellata
Malus x moerlandsii 'Profusion' (CRAB APPLE)
Muscari armeniacum (GRAPE HYACINTH) ★
Narcissus cvs. (many, particularly JONQUILS) ★
Osmanthus delavayi
Populus balsamifera (BALSAM POPLAR)
Primula florindae (PRIMROSE)
Prunus padus (BIRD CHERRY)
Rhododendron luteum (AZALEA)
Spartium junceum (SPANISH BROOM)
Syringa vulgaris CVS. (LILAC)
Viburnum x burkwoodii
Viola odorata (VIOLET)
Wisteria sinensis

Summer

Alyssum maritimum ★
Brunfelsia pauciflora (THORN APPLE)
Buddleja colvilei and *B. fallowiana* var. *alba* (BUTTERFLY BUSH)
Caryopteris x clandonensis (BLUE SPIRAEA)
Cytisus battandieri (PINEAPPLE BROOM)
Deutzia x elegantissima
Dianthus 'Mrs Sinkins' (PINK)
Genista aetnensis (MOUNT ETNA BROOM)
Heliotropium arborescens (HELIOTROPE) ★
Hesperis matronalis (SWEET ROCKET) ★
Iris graminea

Itea ilicifolia
Lathyrus odoratus (SWEET PEA)
Lilium candidum (MADONNA LILY) ★
Lilium regale (REGAL LILY) ★
Lonicera japonica 'Halliana' (HONEYSUCKLE)
Lupinus arboreus (TREE LUPIN)
Magnolia grandiflora
Matthiola bicornis (NIGHT-SCENTED STOCK) ★
Matthiola incana (STOCK) ★
Nicotiana alata, N. sylvestris (TOBACCO PLANT) ★
Perovskia atriplicifolia 'Blue Spire' (RUSSIAN SAGE)
Philadelphus cvs. (MOCK ORANGE BLOSSOM)
Reseda odorata (MIGNONETTE) ★
Robinia pseudoacacia (FALSE ACACIA)
Romneya coulteri (CALIFORNIAN TREE POPPY)
Roses, especially old shrub eg. bourbon
Tilia tomentosa (LIME)
Verbena x hybrida ★

Autumn

Abelia x grandiflora
Ceanothus 'A T Johnson' (CALIFORNIAN LILAC)
Cercidiphyllum japonicum (KATSURA TREE)
Clerodendrum trichotomum
Clethra alnifolia (SWEET PEPPER BUSH)
Elaeagnus x ebbingei
Freesia cvs. ★
Oenothera biennis (EVENING PRIMROSE)
Osmanthus heterophyllus
Phlox paniculata
Rosa rubiginosa (SWEET BRIAR)

Winter

Chimonanthus praecox (WINTER SWEET)
Clematis cirrhosa
Corylopsis sinensis
Daphne mezereum (MEZEREON)
Hamamelis cvs. (WITCH HAZEL)
Iris reticulata and *I. unguicularis* ★
Lonicera fragrantissima (SHRUBBY HONEYSUCKLE)
Mahonia cvs. (OREGON GRAPE)
Sarcococca spp. (CHRISTMAS BOX)
Skimmia japonica
Viburnum farreri, other viburnums

The following have fragrant leaves all year round:
Artemisia 'Powis Castle'
Choisya ternata (MEXICAN ORANGE BLOSSOM)
Cistus x cyprius and *C. x purpureus* (ROCK ROSE)
Myrtus communis (MYRTLE)
Phlomis fruticosa (JERUSALEM SAGE)
Salvia officinalis (SAGE)
Santolina spp. (COTTON LAVENDER)

Uses in the garden

Some plants are useful for more than their healing properties and are worth growing in the garden for their practical benefits. Here are a few ideas:

To mask unpleasant odours, for instance from bins or traffic, the following are natural air fresheners: LEMON, GERANIUM, PEPPERMINT, LAVENDER, CLARY SAGE, CEDARWOOD, JUNIPER, PINE, EUCALYPTUS, THYME, ROSEMARY.

To repel unwanted insects in the garden plant EUCALYPTUS, LAVENDER OR ROSEMARY.

For fragrance while entertaining outside, throw a handful of the following on to a barbecue: ANGELICA SEEDHEADS, LAVENDER FLOWERS, JUNIPER TWIGS AND BRANCHES, LOVAGE SEEDHEADS, PINE CONES, ROSEMARY TWIGS, SAGE LEAVES AND TWIGS, SOUTHERNWOOD TWIGS (*Artemisia abrotanum*).

To refresh hot summer air plant ROSEMARY, PEPPERMINT, BASIL OR GRAPEFRUIT.

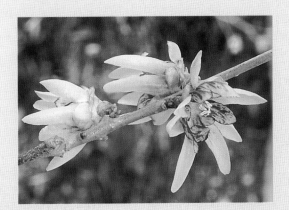

LEFT The common name of *Chimonanthus praecox* is winter sweet, which perfectly describes the fragrance from the delicate flowers that appear on bare stems in the middle of winter.

A relaxing retreat

BELOW The planting
surrounding this seat will
have a doubly relaxing
effect upon anyone sitting
there: the scent from the
massed roses will be
calming, while the soft
colours of lady's mantle
(*Alchemilla mollis*),
foxgloves (*Digitalis
purpurea*) and
sisyrinchium enhance the
peaceful mood.

For obvious reasons, this area should be peaceful and enticing, preferably a little way from the house so that you can escape from everyday distractions. Placed in light shade, the area should offer respite from the heat of the day so that you will be encouraged to sit for a while. Wherever possible, disturbing noise should be masked; consider installing moving water or improving sound insulation through a dense planting screen. Aim to make the spot as quiet and secluded as possible and also give some thought to the outlook from the seat you will place there. The seat should be comfortable, with cushions for a touch of luxury, and if it is possible to lie down, so much the better. You might even wish to erect a hammock, if feasible, so that you can be gently lulled by the swaying motion.

The plants you choose should have restful qualities and could include any of the following: CEDARWOOD, CHAMOMILE, CLARY SAGE, CYPRESS, GERANIUM, HOPS, JUNIPER, LAVENDER, MARJORAM, MELISSA, ROSE, VALERIAN, VIOLET, YARROW.

Other suitable plants would have a sweet, light, floral fragrance which will waft gently over you.

In addition to scent, a very important aspect of such a garden is colour. As we have seen in the chapter on Colour Therapy, the hues at the cooler range of the colour spectrum will encourage relaxation and engender a restful mood. Make use of greens, blues and purples, perhaps moving into pale pinks or yellows, with highlights from touches of white or cream. Such colours help create a harmonious state of mind and work together with the aromas to induce complete relaxation and a balanced mood.

Such a spot presents an ideal opportunity to include a focus for meditation, which will help you switch off more easily (see the next chapter).

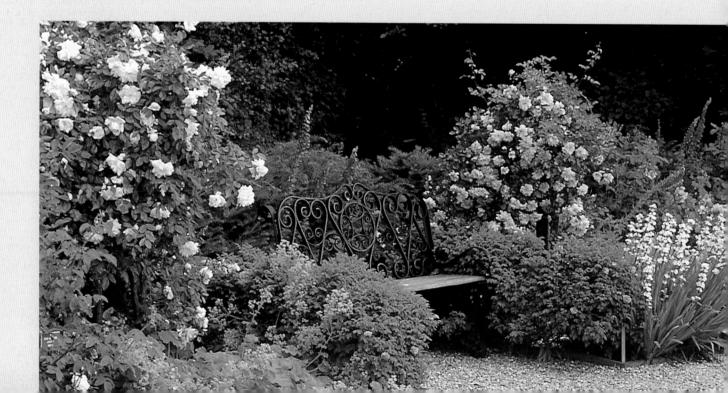

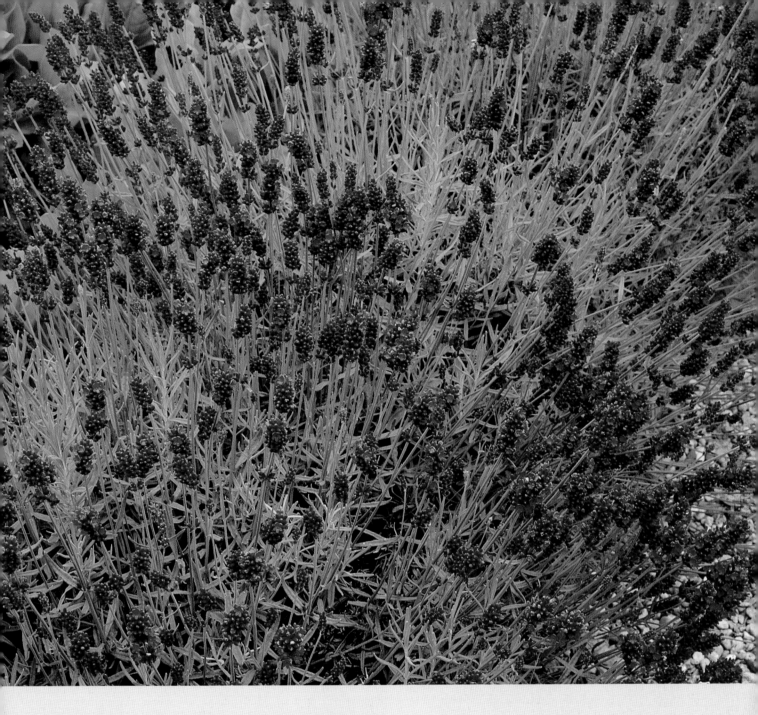

A garden to get you going

If, on the other hand, you need to be invigorated, an entirely different area can be created. Such a spot is best sited to make the most of any sun within the garden so that sitting in it will warm and revitalize you, filling you with energy. On a sunless day, deep breathing of certain stimulating scents will have a similar effect.

The revitalizing garden should contain fragrances from the spicy, woody or citrus range. The plantings might include any of the following, all of which will lift the spirits and fire you with enthusiasm for life: ANGELICA, BASIL, CITRUS, CYPRESS, EUCALYPTUS, FENNEL, GERANIUM, JASMINE, LAVENDER, PEPPERMINT, PINE, ROSE, ROSEMARY, THYME.

Other fragrant plants should have a 'punchy' scent, with refreshing, green undertones or a hint of citrus.

Bright, strong hues will energize you and the warming tones of yellow, orange and red encourage movement and vitality. Such an area offers an ideal opportunity to make use of a full range of annuals, whose brilliant colour will brighten the garden with their ephemeral presence: nasturtium, pot marigold, sunflowers, gazania, salvia and geraniums.

ABOVE The essential oil produced by lavender (*Lavandula angustifolia* 'Hidcote') has a balancing effect, so that it is equally able to uplift and invigorate, or relax.

A lovers' garden

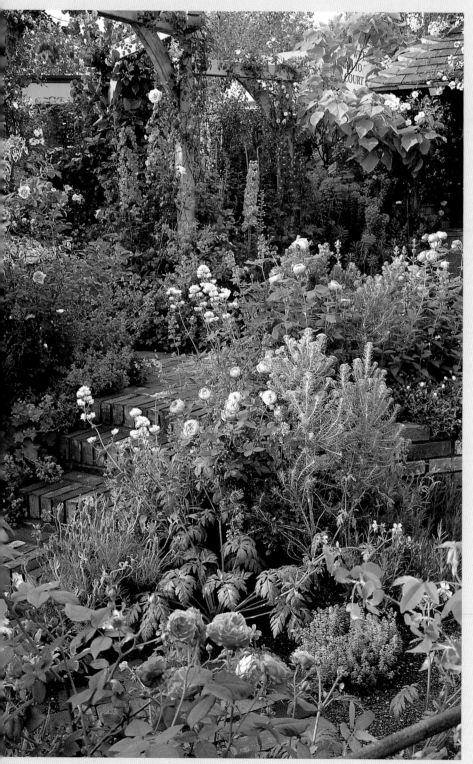

A sensual garden can be created especially for two. Such an area is best placed in a secluded spot, sheltered from everyday intrusions so that a couple can relax and enjoy each other's company, and perhaps share a bottle of wine.

The following mood-enhancing plants will encourage a more loving atmosphere. These aphrodisiac fragrances each have slightly different effects and a mixture of three or four is most effective (preferably selecting one from each appropriate section). It is important that each fragrance is favoured by both parties.

Reducing stress: LAVENDER
Improving confidence: JASMINE or ROSE
Mellowing, encouraging withdrawal from the outside world: CARNATION, CEDARWOOD, CHAMOMILE or MIMOSA
Warming, stimulating: ANGELICA, BASIL, CARNATION, FENNEL or JUNIPER
Energizing or refreshing: CITRUS, GERANIUM, LAVENDER, PEPPERMINT, PINE or ROSEMARY
Improving communication: CLARY SAGE, GERANIUM or ROSE

Suitable colours for this garden would be rich purples and pinks, moving from pale mauves through to deep sultry purples with perhaps an occasional splash of passionate red.

LEFT The sultry tones of pinks, mauves and purples in this garden will create a romantic atmosphere. The roses help open up communication for a more caring relationship, and the French lavender (*Lavandula stoechas*) will reduce stress and balance the emotions.

RIGHT This combination of jasmine (*Jasminum officinale* 'Aureum') and golden hop (*Humulus lupulus* 'Aureus') provides a backdrop for a woman's garden. These plants have a balancing and calming effect and should make a woman feel more attractive; her sex drive might also improve!

A woman's garden

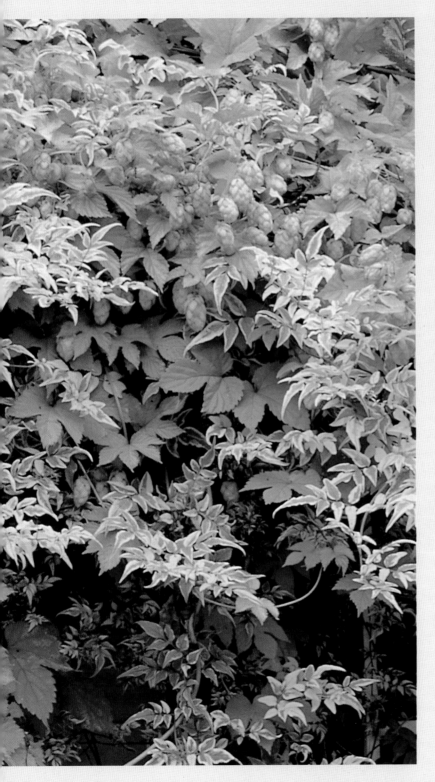

Certain plants have a beneficial effect upon the female reproductive system through their ability to balance hormones. In addition, some plants such as rhubarb, hops, fennel, red clover and sage have been found to contain oestrogen-like substances, which regulate the menstrual cycle and are particularly useful during the menopause as they enhance the body's ability to balance its own hormones.

Relief for the following problems might be found through the creation of an area filled with a selection of suitable plants. Choose three or four that you find appealing and are suited to your garden environment.

Pre-menstrual syndrome includes various physical and emotional symptoms which are brought about by hormonal changes within the body.

Reducing irritability: CHAMOMILE, HOPS
(*if not depressed*) or LAVENDER
Relieving depression: CLARY SAGE
Balancing mood swings: GERANIUM
Reducing feeling of unattractiveness, improving confidence: JASMINE or ROSE
Easing water retention: CLARY SAGE, CYPRESS, FENNEL, JUNIPER or ROSEMARY
Soothing period pains: CHAMOMILE, CLARY SAGE, LAVENDER or MARJORAM

During the menopause, many women suffer a range of symptoms which are again brought about by hormonal imbalance. Some symptoms are the same as those of pre-menstrual syndrome; try the plants listed above, or the following:

Balancing body and mind: HOPS, MELISSA or ROSE
Relieving water retention: FENNEL, JUNIPER or ROSEMARY
Regulating periods: CYPRESS or ROSE
Lessening fatigue: ROSEMARY
Relieving insomnia: LAVENDER or MARJORAM
Improving sex drive: CLARY SAGE, JASMINE or ROSE
Relieving dizziness: PEPPERMINT
Improving concentration: BASIL or PEPPERMINT
Relieving hot flushes: CHAMOMILE or GERANIUM

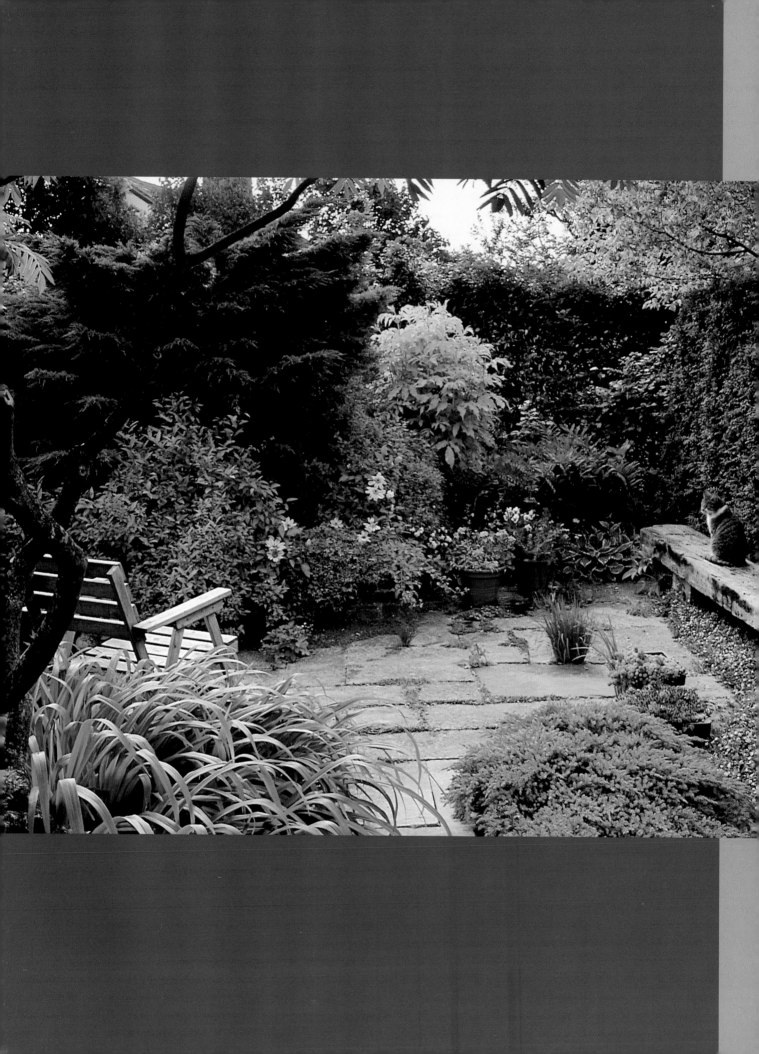

6 Meditation

The kiss of the sun for pardon
The song of the birds for mirth
One is nearer God's Heart in the garden
Than anywhere else on earth.

DOROTHY FRANCES GURNEY

The garden has always been central to our quest for spiritual fulfilment. It offers a retreat from everyday life and provides endless opportunities for relaxation, refreshment and sanctuary. Religious communities have their cloisters and other secluded areas for quiet contemplation, while parks and pleasure gardens provide an enduring image of secular enjoyment. A garden can become our personal haven; it is a place where we can, and should, express ourselves freely, our own small corner of paradise.

Even where little thought or planning has gone into a garden, the simple pleasures of being in close contact with nature are many. Is there anyone who doesn't identify with at least one of the following? The satisfaction of watching a plant grow from seed; watering the garden at the end of a hot day; savouring the fragrance of honeysuckle or the fresh 'green' smell of newly cut grass; relaxing in the sun on a warm summer afternoon; eating an apple straight from the tree, or capturing the fleeting beauty of a flower that wasn't there yesterday and will be gone tomorrow.

The secret is to learn to enjoy gardening and not to regard it grudgingly as yet another chore. We might lead busy lives, but our quest for the 'low maintenance' garden often means that we view routine tasks as millstones around our necks. If we could learn to see our gardens in a different light and actively seek out opportunities for relaxation, we would find literally hundreds. Mowing the grass, weeding, pruning, staking, deadheading; all these simple jobs offer a perfect opportunity to concentrate on the task in hand and free the mind from the everyday worries of work, family and money. Every time we sow seeds, plant bulbs or fill containers and hanging baskets we become aware of the yearly cycle and give ourselves something to look forward to over the coming months. When bad weather prevents us from working in the garden, we can take the opportunity to flick through seed catalogues, read up on garden design, or learn about pruning techniques. By working with the natural rhythm of the seasons, we might find we take pleasure in the needs of our gardens instead of fighting against them.

LEFT A corner of the garden can provide sanctuary from the activity in the remainder of your home.

Stress

Most of us would benefit enormously from learning to relax – both mentally and physically – and our health would be vastly improved if we could do so on a regular basis. As our lives become ever more frenzied, we constantly hear about the perils of 'stress', and many sources now believe that it is the root cause of almost every illness. Evidence suggests that we should all pay more heed to this age-old response to fear and anger, and perhaps start to deal with it more effectively.

When under extreme stress, our body prepares us for action: the 'fight or flight' response. Through a complex interaction between body and mind, a cocktail of adrenaline and other hormones is released, which speeds up our metabolism and raises our pulse and rate of breathing. Blood sugar, insulin and cholesterol levels rise and our digestive and immune systems 'shut down' to allow our bodies to focus on the immediate problem. Natural painkillers, such as cortisone and endorphins, are also released and our senses become heightened. Although poised to take physical action, most of the situations we find ourselves in these days allow us neither to attack the cause of our anguish nor run away! Long-term problems can arise when we are unable to act physically and clear these chemicals from our systems. When we can't react appropriately, stress hormones build up over time, leading to a gradual winding down of our immune system, which leaves us vulnerable to illness.

However, if we learn and practise suitable relaxation techniques, such as meditation, our adrenaline levels fall and potentially dangerous reactions to stress can be successfully defused. This chapter sets out some simple techniques that will aid relaxation, using the garden as a point of reference and source of inspiration.

What is meditation?

During meditation the aim is to reach a state in which the body is relaxed and the mind peaceful, yet alert. Our attention is focused in the present: this is the most beneficial state for healing as we are less likely to be distracted by past or future concerns and can simply concentrate on the here and now.

The power of deep relaxation can be detected via the electrical impulses of the brain, which follow differing rhythms according to our state of wakefulness. Beta brainwaves are rapid and denote an active state of mind, which is associated particularly with the left (logical) side of the brain. Alpha brainwaves are less chaotic and become dominant when we relax and the electrical activity of our mind literally slows down. In the alpha state we become more receptive to our intuitive inner nature. In many ways alpha and beta states have much in common with the principles of *yin* and *yang* (see page 40): we need to experience a balance of both at appropriate times in order to be in harmony with ourselves. During the day, we constantly (and unwittingly) switch between these states, each suiting different tasks. Through meditation we can learn to alter our thought patterns from active to passive and thus adjust our mindset in order to bring about controlled healing. Two other brain states exist – theta and delta – that denote light and deeper sleep patterns. Neither of these is encountered in meditation, the intention being not to 'drop off' but to retain an aware, albeit tranquil, state of mind.

The basic stages in meditation are to relax, to choose a suitable focus and then to let go of everything else in your mind. Obviously this is much easier said than done but, like most things, it does become simpler with practice and you should soon start to become aware of improvements in your health, both mental and physical. The release of tension brings about increased physical and mental energy, improved concentration, freedom from anxiety, better sleep, inner peace, and the ability to face challenges and see things in a positive light. Some find meditation difficult initially as it often makes us feel vulnerable; we may fear a loss of control as we let go and become more aware of our inner thoughts and emotional responses. If you find that this is the case, it may be advisable to join an organized class in order to get to grips with the finer points of the art.

Most people find that relaxation is easier to achieve when something holds the attention and the mind is focused to prevent it constantly drifting back to everyday thoughts and worries. One way of maintaining concentration is to meditate upon a subject; this may be a tangible object such as a statue, candle, tree or flower, or something more abstract such as a pattern of breathing, a repeated word or phrase (mantra) or mental image. Choose a technique that appeals to you and an object, if appropriate, that you find attractive. If you find it hard to concentrate on something static, it can be equally constructive to watch nature at work – the passing of clouds or birds in the sky, colours in a beautiful sunrise or sunset, swirling patterns of water in a stream, grass moving in the wind, or falling rain.

It is theoretically possible to meditate in any posture, although the options are slightly more limited in the garden. The only requirements are that you feel comfortable and are able to breathe freely. Breathing technique is important, but it is enough to breathe slowly and evenly at all times, concentrating on making the out breath longer than the in breath.

Some find the practice of yoga or *tai ch'i* aids concentration, and carefully selected background music can also be beneficial (as long as it is acceptable to your neighbours).

You can meditate at any time of the day, whenever you have the time, although you may need to be adaptable to work around the changing weather in the garden. For many, the best time is either first thing in the morning, before they start the day, or in the evening after work. To achieve optimum results, aim to set aside a minimum of fifteen minutes each day. We all need to slow down in order to recharge our batteries and this resting time is essential to the process of healing, both physically and spiritually. During this time, learn to see every feature of your garden as if through new eyes. Free yourself from everyday worries and simply appreciate the moment, regardless of whatever else is going on in your life. Through this new appreciation of your surroundings you will soon feel the benefits of connecting with your mental and emotional self.

Healing meditation

Meditation can reconnect us with our inner energies, which have a vital role to play in the natural healing process. As an holistic practice, meditation harmonizes the entire person. It encourages us to keep in touch with the sensations of our bodies and minds, so we can more easily learn to recognize early signs of illness and work on them before they develop into something more serious.

Meditation and relaxation assist natural healing through a range of physical improvements, which include the following:

- a better flow of blood to parts of the body that are deprived in times of stress (particularly the skin, brain and digestive system);
- opening up of the airways, which improves circulation and is of particular benefit to asthmatics and hay fever sufferers;
- balancing of hormonal activity, which is adversely affected by the build-up of adrenaline (particularly beneficial for those suffering infertility);
- lowering of blood pressure; release of muscular tension to ease aches and pains;
- stimulation of the immune system, which is less efficient during times of stress.

These improvements, and others, are also helpful for sufferers of insomnia, tension headaches and migraine, pre-menstrual syndrome, mild depression, chronic pain and allergies, irritable bowel syndrome, and during convalescence.

Although powerful on its own, meditation is probably most effective when used to support a cure (through either allopathic or complementary means) rather than to bring one about by itself. Relaxation techniques have been found to be very valuable **alongside** the conventional treatment of cancer, AIDS, heart problems and other life-threatening conditions.

Even if it cannot bring about a cure, meditation will almost certainly help you to deal better with your problems and also the side effects of any treatment you may be receiving.

Meditation in the garden

Many gardens are naturally calming places and provide a sanctuary in which to recover from stress. Our gardens can also refresh us spiritually and it is possible to create a structured setting for meditation through the incorporation of certain features. The aim of these is to aid relaxation and provide a focus for concentration, which will enhance the healing experience. Bear in mind that your garden is, above all, a source of enjoyment, so aim only to satisfy your own particular needs and choose the element(s) that fit your personal requirements.

To create a garden setting appropriate to contemplation, the simpler the layout, the better. You might consider designs based on circles (representing the cycle of life and the seasons), squares (denoting universal order), or symbols such as the Celtic knot (which represents a journey). Avoid clashing colours and a cluttered layout; these will grab your attention and distract your concentration. Simplicity is the key to establishing an air of tranquillity.

Water

Possibly the most valuable component of the meditation garden is water. Water is a perfect focal point for contemplation, either in the form of a still, reflective pool or a fountain or gentle waterfall.

Bear in mind that the shape and style of a pool should reflect the character of the garden: use symmetrical shapes in a formal garden and a more curvaceous outline for an informal feel. In *feng shui* (see Chapter 2), a flat sheet of water is considered an important complement to the vertical elements of the garden, thereby achieving a balance of *yin* and *yang*. Even in a very small garden, a water feature could consist of a Japanese-style stone basin (see picture, page 157) or a wooden tub, either of which could be planted with miniature water lilies (*Nymphaea pygmaea*) from a specialist garden centre. Moving water is also valuable as long as it has a gentle presence and is not a gushing torrent! Again, possibilities for smaller gardens include flowforms, similar to that pictured on page 30.

Seating

In order to relax totally and concentrate on meditation, many people choose to sit or lie down; if you have a suitable area of grass, this may be all that is required. However, if you need a little more comfort or want to use the garden in all seasons, a seat of some type will be helpful. Any garden seat is appropriate as long as it is comfortable enough to encourage you to sit for a reasonable length of time. Add cushions to a hard chair or bench if necessary, but remember that the aim is not to fall asleep! The gentle swaying of a hammock is very relaxing, but it offers little support to the body and may impede deep breathing if you slump too much.

The location of your seating is important. If any object in the garden is to be used as a focus for concentration, the seat should face it directly so that your head does not have to be turned to afford a clear view. Full, bright sunlight makes concentration difficult, while dense shade will not entice you to spend time there and will feel dank and gloomy at many times of the year. For these reasons, either position the seat in light shade or dappled sunlight or set up some kind of canopy; this would also enable you to use the garden when it is raining.

Alternatively, you may prefer to wander slowly around the garden, always remembering to breathe slowly and evenly. Pay close attention to the individual leaves and flowers you come across and try to find something new each time. You will then discover the miraculous changes taking place throughout the seasons and will feel more in harmony with the natural course of things.

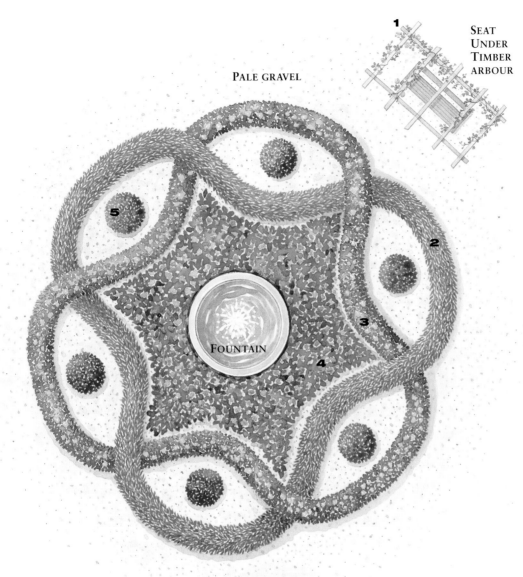

1 SEAT UNDER TIMBER ARBOUR

PALE GRAVEL

FOUNTAIN

1 CLIMBING ROSE (*Rosa 'Veilchenblau'*) AND CLIMBING CLEMATIS (*Clematis viticella 'Etoile Violette'*)

2 LAVENDER (*Lavandula angustifolia 'Hidcote'*)

3 COTTON LAVENDER (*Santolina pinnata subsp. neapolitana 'Edward Bowles'*)

4 VINCA MINOR 'ATROPURPUREA' OR VIOLA RIVINIANA PURPUREA GROUP

5 CLIPPED BOX BALLS *Buxus sempervirens 'Suffruticosa'*

A pattern for thought

A garden in which to relax and meditate; its seat is sheltered and shaded from the sun beneath an arbour clothed with violet-flowering climbers from early summer through to autumn. The fragrance of the rose will also have a calming influence. The silver foliage of lavender and cotton lavender creates a simple yet intriguing pattern, with long-lasting summer flowers in violet and yellow (violet's complementary colour – see Chapter 3, Colour therapy). Violet, an important meditative colour, is also provided at different times of year by ground-cover plantings of *Vinca minor* or *Viola riviniana* 'Purpurea', while the clipped box balls create a sense of rhythm.

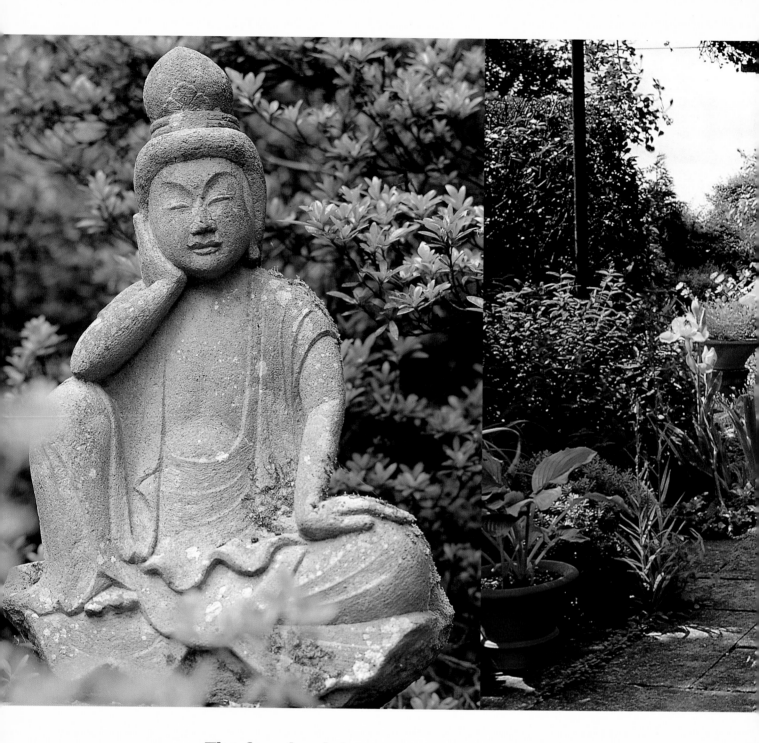

The focal point

You may like to include an object that will provide a focus for meditation and help to keep your attention. This could be a beautiful piece of sculpture or any item of particular significance to you. You might choose to plant a favourite tree or shrub – possibly in a place that holds special memories for you. Although it is often advisable to match the style of an object to the overall scale and character of the garden, never feel bound by convention. All gardens benefit from an element of surprise and if a humorous addition helps to lift your spirits every time you see it, by all means make use of it.

Place any contemplative object against a background that will not distract the eye, such as a fine-textured plant, plain fence or wall. If possible, also contrast the colour of the feature with that of the backdrop so that the outline is clear and the eye does not have to work hard to pick out its shape.

Install some lighting if you intend to use the garden at night; this will add another dimension and can create a magical setting for relaxation.

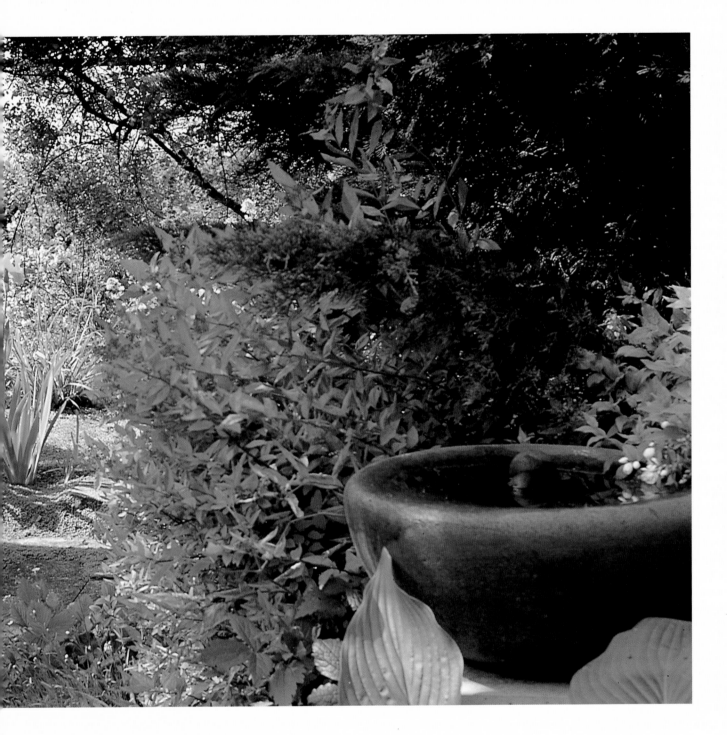

Meditative colours

We have already seen the profound effect that certain colours can have upon both our bodies and minds (see Chapter 3, Colour Therapy). Obviously some colours are better suited to meditation than others and although we each have individual requirements for specific health problems, there are a few general guidelines for meditation areas. The warmer colours of the spectrum such as red, orange and strong yellow tend to encourage activity and are therefore unsuitable for relaxation. Cool colours, with their ability to calm and soothe the senses, are more appropriate and the bulk of the colour from plants and other garden materials should ideally fall within the violet/blue/green range. Violet is a particularly good colour for meditation, being closely linked to the mind and creative visualization.

There is also a place for softer colours in the white, cream, and pale yellow range as these will lend a tranquil mood. Choose plants not only for their colours, but also because you feel drawn to their other qualities: of shape, texture or fragrance.

ABOVE A simple bowl, brimming with water, might fit your own requirements better than a figurative form; it could also serve as a birdbath, rewarding you with the pleasure of visiting wildlife.

157

Visualization

The technique of visualization can be used to hold the attention in place of a defined focus. It entails placing yourself in a fictitious scenario and using your imagination to experience it physically, mentally and emotionally. Ideally, all five senses are involved: sight, scent, sound, touch and taste should be included in the imagery. When practised effectively, visualization leaves you feeling relaxed and positive.

The most beneficial visualizations are often very personal; you imagine yourself in a place you would like to be. It might be on a faraway beach, at a happy occasion with close family and friends, or anywhere that holds good memories for you. Even your own garden can provide wonderful imagery; envisage yourself relaxing on a perfect summer day, with the grass mown and the borders weeded and only birdsong and the hum of insects to disturb you. The technique is simple: clear the mind of other thoughts, relax and close your eyes so that you can let your imagination take over. If you find it difficult to find a source of ideas, the following might be helpful. You could ask a friend to read it to you or make a tape of yourself reading it.

Imagine yourself sitting on a chair in the living room of a beautiful old house. You catch a glimpse of the lovely gardens through an open door and you stand up and walk towards it for a better view. You reach the door and become aware of the heat of the summer's day. You step down into the garden. Your feet are bare and you feel the warmth of the flagstones through your soles; this warmth slowly spreads through your whole body.

You walk towards a lawn and, stepping on to it, you feel the softness and coolness of the grass, the springy stems bending under your feet. Walk slowly across the grass, feeling the warmth of the sun on every part of your body. You can smell the sweet

scents of summer roses and all is quiet but for the trees rustling in the light, refreshing breeze and a little birdsong. You pass a strawberry bush and bend down to pick a fruit from it. Taste the flesh as it fills your mouth with its aromatic sweetness, the juice refreshing your throat as you swallow.

In the distance you can just hear trickling water. Start walking towards the sound, enjoying the warmth, sounds and smells of the summer's day. You turn a corner and see a fountain; the sun is glinting off the water and it looks cool and inviting so you walk over to it. Sitting down on the edge of the fountain, feel the coolness of the stones against your body. Run your hands gently through the water, allowing the drops to splash against your skin as you feel yourself cooling down. There is bright green moss growing over the stonework; feel its thick velvet texture as you run your fingers over it.

When you feel quite cool, you slowly get up and begin to walk back towards the house. The sun is still hot, the garden quiet and fragrant; you stop and lie down on some grass. Just lie there for a while feeling the soft springiness supporting your body and the warmth of the sun on your face.

After a while you slowly stand up and start walking back to the path. Step on to the path and feel the warmth of the stones again in contrast to the coolness of the grass. Walk up the path and, passing a lavender bush, breathe in the scent that is released as you brush against its leaves. Continue slowly back to the door that you first came through. Stepping up from the path through the door, you pass into the cool and refreshing room; go to the chair and sit down, and simply savour the experiences of the garden for a few moments longer.

When you feel ready, slowly bring yourself back to reality, open your eyes and gently stretch your body.

Zen gardens

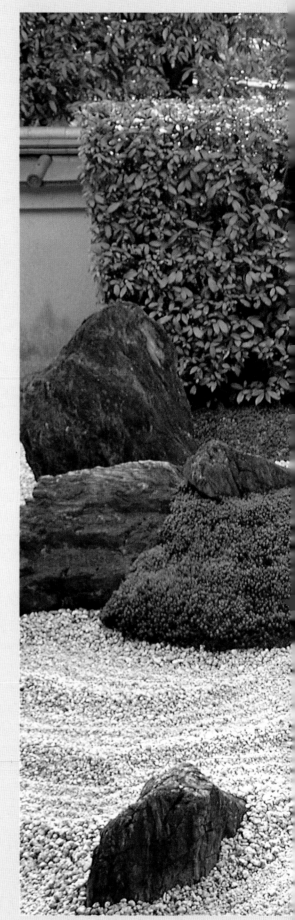

The ultimate meditation gardens might be considered to be the Zen gravel gardens of Japan, in which the minimalist approach has been taken to the limit in order to avoid unwanted distraction. The placement of every plant, stone and feature is afforded absolute attention to detail and we could learn much from the fine art of such gardens in our pursuit of harmony.

While the representation of paradise is a common thread running through gardens around the world, Oriental gardens have always attempted this in an entirely different manner from gardens in the West. Throughout history, Western gardeners have striven to tame the wilder aspects of nature and extend their power over the natural world. Meanwhile, Shinto and Taoist beliefs have always delighted in the beauty of nature. Followers of Zen Buddhism believe that the attainment of a blissful state is possible only when there is a balance of *yin* and *yang*, whether in the form of trees, rocks and water or qualities such as light and shade, shape and texture. Oriental gardens are, for the most part, strongly symbolic, and the principle of harmony is of the utmost importance.

Zen Buddhism has existed in Japan since the tenth century and slowly evolved as Japanese priests returned from China, not only with new religious ideas but also impressions of various art forms. Over time, artists began to experiment in more diverse fields such as garden-making, which they originally based on what they had seen in China. Using the raw materials of rocks and sand, they made 'paintings' to create an evocative impression of a landscape, every rock being carefully selected and meticulously placed to represent specific features. These *karesansui*, or 'dry landscape' gardens were, and are, primarily works of art and gardens second.

By the sixteenth century, the same materials were being used to portray a conceptualized vision of the universe, or nature as a whole; a new style of garden

RIGHT The Zen garden is typified by this careful composition of rocks, gravel and a few immaculately tended plants at the Ryoan-ji temple, Kyoto, Japan.

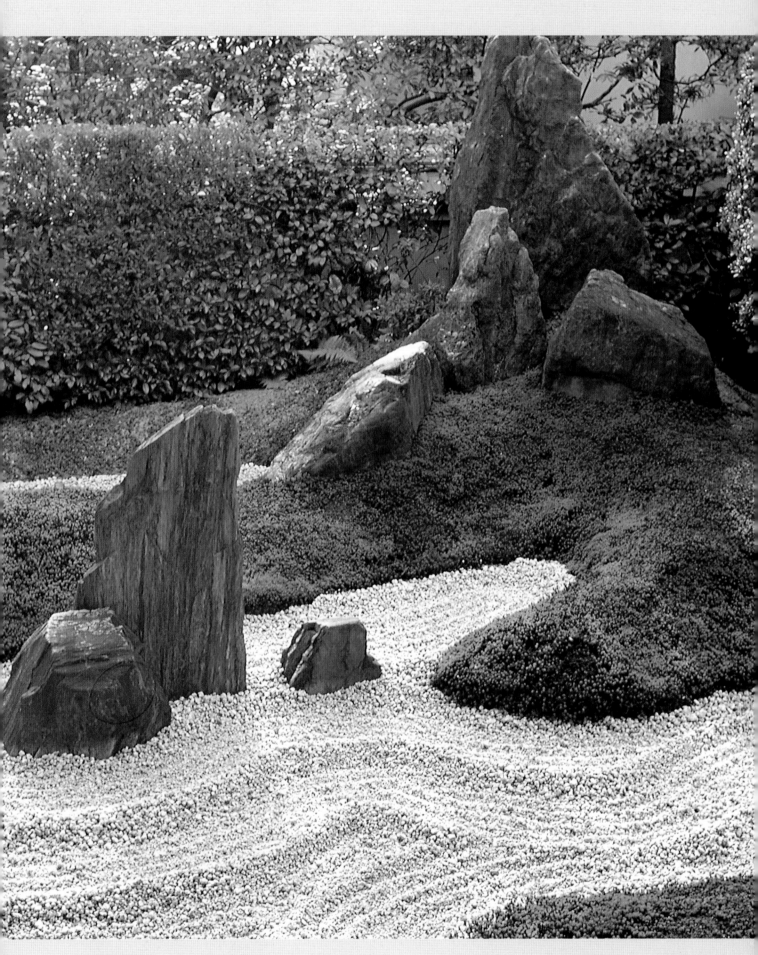

had developed. Such gardens evolved to satisfy the Zen priests' spiritual and aesthetic needs for a setting that was appropriate to their silent contemplation. The gardens were designed to be viewed at close quarters from inside a building during long bouts of meditation. Traditionally, the Zen garden was contained within walls or screens. Through the contrived use of materials, the Japanese found they could represent nature in a confined space and bring the symbolism of mountains and rivers into the garden. The forms of the elements of stones, plants and space was dominant. Colour played a minor role so that it didn't distract the attention and subtle textural contrasts were brought about through the use of foliage, moss, stone, gravel and water. The aim was always to soothe the eye and achieve balance, movement and variation.

Today, Zen gardens contain three principal elements: rocks, water and plants – and of these, stone probably has the most important role. Some Zen gardens contain very little else and rely mainly upon the inherent qualities of the rocks and the skill of composition for interest. Individual rocks and stones are revered for their shape, colour or texture and are laid out according to the 'principle of three forces'. This is derived from Chinese painting and comprises vertical, horizontal and diagonal lines – representing the Heavens, Earth and Man. Vertical lines establish depth, horizontal lines stability, and diagonal lines provide a link between the other two, easing the transition.

Individual rocks are chosen to exhibit one or two such characteristics and are then carefully positioned to form a triangle, in both plan and elevation. The composition should appear stable, yet dynamic. The rocks are also placed so that any lines of strata appear in the same plane as they would have occurred originally or when found.

One very popular stone grouping is the *sanzon*, where three stones are placed with the tallest at the centre, to represent Buddha and two of his attendants. Two important symbols of longevity and good fortune are often represented – the turtle (*kame*) and crane (*tsuru*). In a grouping known as

tsurukame, stones are used to symbolize this pair; horizontal to denote the turtle and vertical for the crane. Through such arrangements, the garden is intended to have a positive and meaningful influence upon the viewer.

Soil is occasionally mounded gently to create the illusion of 'hills' in the background and weathered stone may be used to represent distant mountains. Both are carefully placed so that the design is as naturalistic as possible. A dry riverbed is often represented by flat rocks, to give the impression that water might one day flow again; gravel and pebbles may be used to give the illusion of dry streams. Sand or gravel, when raked into patterns, denotes flowing water or the sea. The act of raking pebbles or sand was considered an element of meditation and is in itself very relaxing.

Water is believed to purify the spirit and even its suggestion in the garden is a valuable tool that can be put to good use where water itself is not a viable option (for instance where there are young children). The belief that water might be present is often enough to bring harmony to a design. Where it is used in the garden, the ideal is to strike a balance between motion – a *yang* force – and stillness, which is considered to be more *yin*. There are many examples of *tsukubai* (water basin) or similar features that can be included in such gardens, many requiring very little space.

Features such as *tsukubai* and *ishi-toro* (stone lanterns) have crept into Japanese gardens over time through the evolution of the tea garden. This development occurred in response to a practical need to maintain the monks' concentration during prolonged periods of meditation. The tea ceremony became central to the design of such gardens, although elements such as stone lanterns, wash basins and stepping stones are not normally found in a true Zen garden. However, if they suit your requirements and you feel they help you achieve the look you are after, make use of them and don't torture yourself over their authenticity – at the end of the day it is your garden, to be planned however you wish.

RIGHT Although not entirely appropriate in the most disciplined Zen garden, this water feature adds elements of sound and movement to an otherwise still landscape. Simple to construct and install, such a device would fit even the tiniest of gardens.

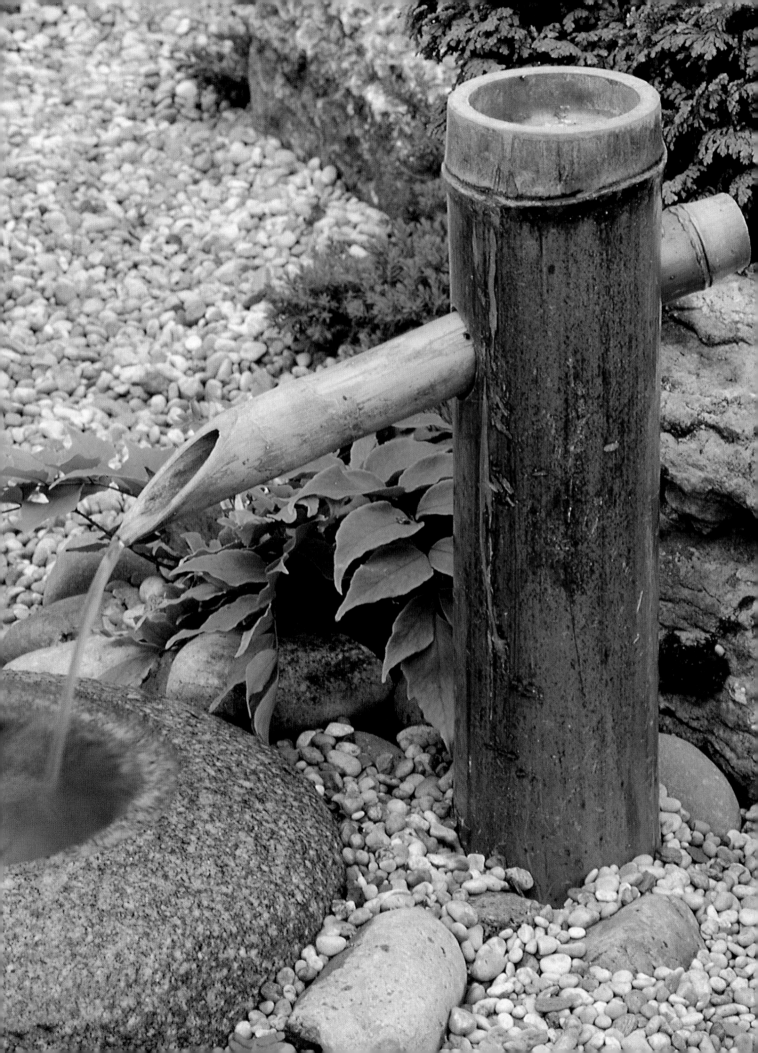

Designing a zen garden

To create a garden that appears harmonious, keep your objectives in mind at all times during the planning process. Try to avoid particularly busy, noisy or exposed areas, which will inevitably be distracting. A Zen garden can be constructed in a tiny space, such as a courtyard, or can make up part of a larger garden. You simply need a regular-shaped area that is fairly open and not hemmed in by overhanging deciduous trees (or you will be raking leaves from your gravel for many weeks of the year).

Zen gardens are normally designed to be viewed from a fixed point and are not to be used in any practical sense as this would ruin their sense of scale and perspective. The impression of a larger natural landscape is created through the precise manipulation of size, texture and colour. Carefully placed stones represent long-distance views and introduce rhythm into the composition, while plants such as azaleas may be pruned to represent a backdrop of far-off mountains. To maintain the illusion of a deeper perspective, bold-textured plants are used in the foreground with finer-leafed varieties in the background. Similarly, stronger colours are placed to the fore and more muted tones to the rear

Most Zen gardens are at least partially enclosed and the prime consideration is the position from which the garden will most often be viewed. This might be from part of the house or from another point in the garden. Wherever possible, aim to retain glimpses of scenery beyond the boundaries – this is the principle of *shakkei* (borrowed landscape), which is an important feature of Japanese gardens. The integrity of the garden will be maintained if you use traditional materials such as split bamboo for fencing, although red-brick walls and panel fences can be made to look more authentic by painting them a subtle grey or green (or even black) to blend with their surroundings.

Above all else, a Zen garden is designed to be a peaceful place that is particularly suitable for meditation; however, every space will be unique, due to the setting and your own personal requirements. The limited ingredients and restrained planting make it a garden style that requires the absolute minimum of attention – one that is ideally suited to today's busy and pressured lifestyle.

Japanese-style plants

When planning a Zen garden, the principle to bear in mind is always 'less is more'; if you are a true plantsperson at heart and crave a verdant environment, Zen gardens are probably not for you. The concept provides little opportunity for horticultural diversity and your plant selection needs to be restrained to say the least.

Colour and variety are not your priorities; far more important are contrasts between the textures and forms of the plants. Your plant selection should consist primarily of evergreens to provide a constant backdrop, with seasonal highlights from flowering plants such as azaleas or camellia. Select only flowering plants that have strong seasonal associations such as spring flowering cherries and wisteria and use them with restraint. The Japanese do not mass flowers together but use them as individual elements to enhance the overall design. In

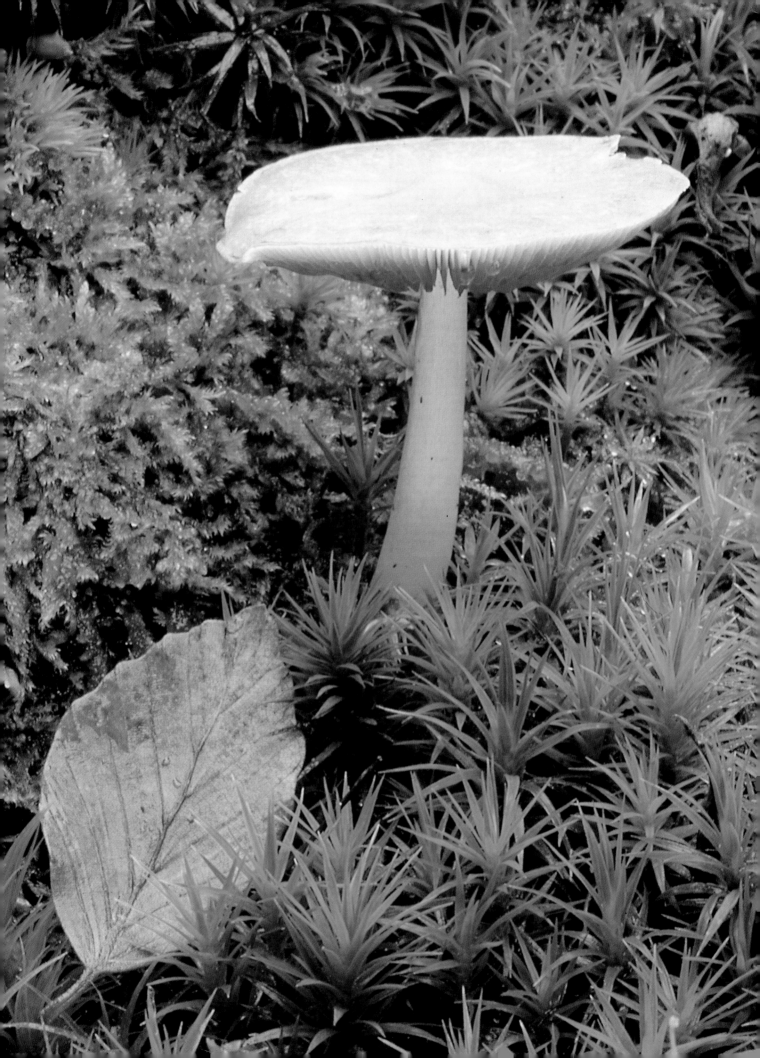

general, colour is regarded as a distraction and the only season where it is traditionally appropriate is autumn; if you include Japanese maples, you will more than make up for the muted tones of the remaining seasons.

The following plants, although not entirely authentic, would lend an appropriate Japanese atmosphere to the garden. Choose selectively!

BELOW Evergreen conifers (firs, cedars and pines) provide a useful backdrop in most Japanese gardens and, in much the same way as *bonsai*, are often pruned so they attain desirable shapes and the appearance of maturity.

Trees

Abies koreana (KOREAN FIR)

Acer palmatum and *A. palmatum* 'Senkaki' (JAPANESE MAPLES)

Cercidiphyllum japonicum (KATSURA TREE)

Cercis siliquastrum (JUDAS TREE)

Cryptomeria japonica (JAPANESE CEDAR)

Ginkgo biloba (MAIDENHAIR TREE)

Magnolia spp.

Paulownia tomentosa (FOXGLOVE TREE)

Pinus parviflora (JAPANESE WHITE PINE)

Pinus thunbergii (JAPANESE BLACK PINE)

Prunus mume (JAPANESE APRICOT)

Prunus subhirtella 'Autumnalis' (AUTUMN CHERRY)

Prunus x yedoensis (YOSHINO CHERRY)

Shrubs and climbers

Amelanchier lamarckii (SNOWY MESPILUS)

Aucuba japonica (LAUREL)

Berberis thunbergii and *Berberis candidula* (BARBERRY)

Buxus sempervirens and *B. sempervirens* 'Suffruticosa' (BOX)

Camellia sasanqua and other varieties (CAMELLIAS)

Chaenomeles japonica and *C. speciosa* (JAPANESE QUINCE)

Daphne odora

Enkianthus campanulatus

Euonymus japonicus

Fargesia murieliae and *F. nitida* (BAMBOO)

Fatsia japonica (FALSE CASTOR OIL PLANT)

Fothergilla major

Hamamelis mollis (WITCH HAZEL)

Hebe albicans (SHRUBBY VERONICA)

Hydrangea anomala subsp. *petiolaris* (CLIMBING HYDRANGEA)

Juniperus sabina 'Tamariscifolia' (PROSTRATE JUNIPER)

Kerria japonica (BACHELORS' BUTTONS)

Mahonia japonica and *M. x media* 'Charity' (OREGON GRAPE)

Nandina domestica (SACRED BAMBOO)

Osmanthus x burkwoodii

Paeonia delavayi and *P. lutea* var. *ludlowii* (TREE PEONIES)

Phyllostachys bambusoides (BAMBOO)

Phyllostachys nigra (BLACK BAMBOO)

Pleioblastus auricomus (BAMBOO)

Pyracantha cvs. (FIRETHORN)

Rhododendron vars.

Skimmia japonica

Spiraea 'Arguta'

Spiraea japonica 'Nana'

Wisteria sinensis (CHINESE WISTERIA)

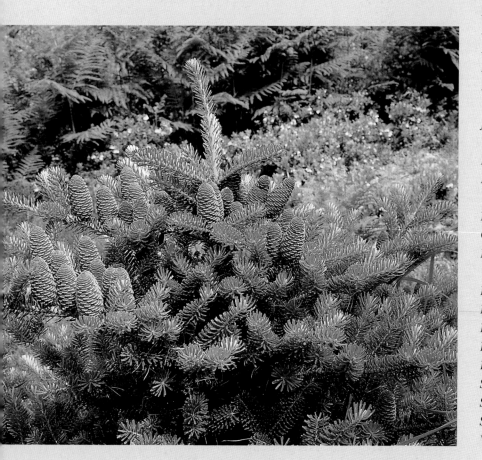

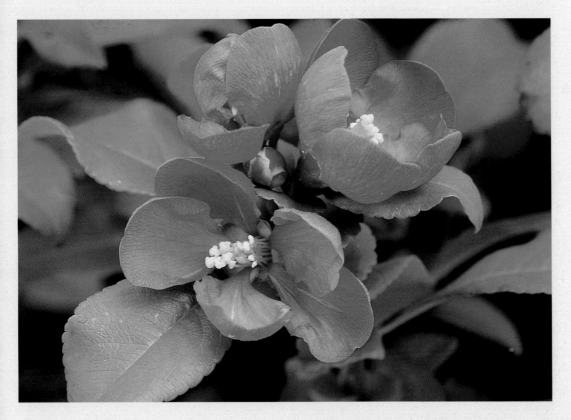

LEFT The Japanese quince is easily grown in most gardens, and provides colour in early spring; *Chaenomeles speciosa* 'Simonii' is relatively low-growing, with semi-double, blood-red flowers.

BELOW *Iris siberica* is a tall, dainty iris available in a range of colours, from the blue type through purples, pinks and white. Although it associates well with water, it grows happily in any moisture-retentive soil.

Herbaceous

Asplenium scolopendrium (MAIDENHAIR FERN)

Athyrium felix-femina (LADY FERN)

Blechnum spicant (HARD FERN)

Festuca eskia and *F. glauca* (BLUE GRASSES)

Hemerocallis fulva (DAY LILY)

Hosta cvs. (PLANTAIN LILY)

Iris ensata and *Iris sibirica* (SIBERIAN IRIS)

Miscanthus sinensis

Molinia caerula

Nerine bowdenii

Platycodon grandiflorus (CHINESE BALLOON
 FLOWER)

Polystichum setiferum 'Pulcherrimum'
 (HARD SHIELD FERN)

Ground cover

Acaena buchananii (NEW ZEALAND BURR)

Bergenia cordifolia (ELEPHANTS' EARS)

Cotoneaster dammeri

Epimedium cvs.

Liriope muscari (TURF LILY)

Mosses

Pinus mugo var. *pumilio* (DWARF MOUNTAIN PINE)

Vinca minor (LESSER PERIWINKLE)

Sasa veitchii (BAMBOO)

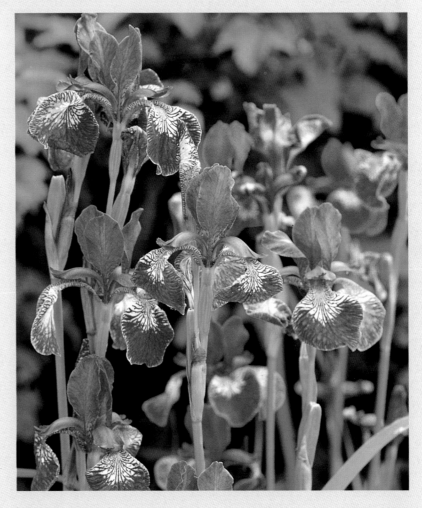

167

Addresses for further information

INTRODUCTION

British Holistic Medical
Association
RT House, Royal Shrewsbury
Hospital South, Shrewsbury
SHROPSHIRE SY3 8XF

HOLISTIC GARDENING

Henry Doubleday Research
Association
Ryton Gardens,
Ryton-on-Dunsmore,
COVENTRY CV8 3LG
(organic gardening)

Soil Association
86 Colston Street,
Bristol AVON BS1 5BB
(organic gardening)

Royal Society for Nature
Conservation
The Green, Witham Park,
Waterside South,
Lincoln LN5 7JR
(encouraging wildlife)

Royal Society for the
Protection of Birds
The Lodge, Sandy
BEDS SG19 2DL
(encouraging birds)

Butterfly Conservation
PO Box 222, Dedham,
Colchester ESSEX CO7 6EY

John Chambers
15 Westleigh Road, Barton
Seagrave, Kettering
NORTHANTS NN15 5AJ
(wildflower seeds and plants)

National Asthma Campaign
Providence House,
Providence Place
LONDON N1 0NT
(support and information)

Probus Gardens
Probus, Truro
CORNWALL TR2 4HQ
(asthma garden display)

FENG SHUI

Feng Shui Network
International
P O Box 2133
LONDON W1A 1RL
(advice and registered
consultants)

Feng Shui World
18 Alacross Road,
LONDON W5 4HT
(consultations)

COLOUR THERAPY

The Hygieia College of
Colour Therapy
Brook House, Avening,
Tetbury GLOS GL8 8NS

The Oracle School of Colour
9 Wyndale Avenue, Kingsbury
LONDON NW9 9PT
(advice and registered
therapists)

HERBALISM

The National Institute of
Medical Herbalists
56 Longbrook Street, Exeter
DEVON EX4 6AH
(registered therapists)

The Society of Homoeopaths
2 Artizan Road,
Northampton
NORTHANTS NN1 4HU
(registered therapists)

Register of Chinese Herbalism
P O Box 400, Wembley
MIDDX HA9 9NZ

Mail order suppliers of herbal
plants (UK and some export):
Salley Gardens
32 Lansdowne Drive, West
Bridgford NOTTS NG2 7FJ

Arne Herbs
Limeburn Nurseries,
Limeburn Hill, Chew Magna
AVON BS18 8QW

Barwinnock Herbs
Barrhill, by Girvan, Ayrshire
SCOTLAND KA26 0RB

Grange Cottage Herbs
4 Grange Cottages
Nailstone, Nuneaton
WARKS CV13 0QN

Jekka's Herb Farm
Rose Cottage
Shellards Lane
Alveston
Bristol AVON BS12 2SY

The Dr Edward Bach Centre
Mount Vernon
Sotwell
Wallingford
OXON OX10 0PZ
(Bach Flower Remedies
information)

AROMATHERAPY

International Federation of
Aromatherapists
Stamford House
2–4 Chiswick High Road
LONDON W4 1TH
(advice and registered
therapists)

International Society of
Professional Aromatherapists
82 Ashby Road
Hinckley
LEICS LE10 1SN
(advice and registered
therapists)

The Register of Qualified
Aromatherapists
P O Box 6491
LONDON N8 9HF

MEDITATION

British Wheel of Yoga
Central Office
1 Hamilton Place
Boston Road
Sleaford
LINCS NG34 7ES
(advice and details of classes)

The Mind Body and Music Co
4 Forester Road
Bath
AVON BA2 6QF

Japanese Garden Society
Honorary Secretary
Groves Mill
Shakers Lane
Long Itchington
WARWICKSHIRE
CV23 8QB

Suggested reading

GENERAL

The RHS Plant Finder
(Dorling Kindersley, updated
annually)

*The RHS Gardeners'
Encyclopedia of Plants and
Flowers,*
Ed. Christopher Brickell
(Dorling Kindersley, 1989)

INTRODUCTION

The Natural Year
Jane Alexander (Bantam
Books, 1997)

The Bodymind Workbook
Debbie Shapiro (Element
Books, 1990)

Managing Stress
Ursula Markham (Element
Books, 1989)

*The Hamlyn Encyclopedia of
Complementary Health*
Ed. Nikki Bradford (Hamlyn,
1996)

HOLISTIC GARDENING

*The Complete Manual of
Organic Gardening*
Basil Caplan (Headline Book
Publishing, 1993)

Successful Organic Gardening
Geoff Hamilton (Dorling
Kindersley, 1987)

*The RHS Book of Pests &
Diseases*
Pippa Greenwood (Dorling
Kindersley, 1997)

*How to Make a Wildlife
Garden*
Chris Baines (Elm Tree
Books, 1986)

*Attracting Birds to Your
Garden*
Stephen Moss and David
Cottridge (New Holland
Publishers, 1998)

*Creating a Low-Allergen
Garden*
Lucy Huntington (Mitchell
Beazley, 1998)

Creative Vegetable Gardening
Joy Larkcom (Mitchell
Beazley, 1997)

FENG SHUI

Feng Shui Made Easy
William Spear (Thorsons,
1995)

The Feng Shui Handbook
Master Lam Kam Chuen
(Gaia Books, 1995)

*The Complete Illustrated
Guide to Feng Shui*
Lillian Too (Element Books,
1996)

COLOUR THERAPY

The Book of Colour Healing
Theo Gimbel (Gaia Books,
1994)

*Reflexology and Colour
Therapy*
Pauline Wills (Element Books,
1992)

Colour in Your Garden
Penelope Hobhouse (Collins,
1985)

*The Gardener's Book of
Colour*
Andrew Lawson (Frances
Lincoln, 1996)

HERBALISM

The Complete Floral Healer
Anne McIntyre (Gaia Books,
1996)

*The Encyclopedia of
Medicinal Plants*
Andrew Chevalier (Dorling
Kindersley, 1996)

*The Encyclopedia of Healing
Plants*
Chrissie Wildwood (Piatkus,
1998)

The Complete Book of Herbs
Lesley Bremness (Dorling
Kindersley, 1988)

Gardening with Herbs
John Stevens (Collins &
Brown, 1996)

*A Handbook of Chinese
Healing Herbs*
Daniel Reid (Simon &
Schuster, 1995)

Good Enough to Eat
Jekka McVicar (Kyle Cathie,
1997)

AROMATHERAPY

*Encyclopedia of
Aromatherapy*
Chrissie Wildwood
(Bloomsbury, 1996)

The Art of Aromatherapy
Robert Tisserand (Arkana,
1977)

*Aromatherapy for Healing the
Spirit*
Gabriel Mojay (Gaia Books,
1996)

The Fragrant Pharmacy and
The Fragrant Mind
Valerie Ann Worwood (both
Bantam Books, 1990 and 1995)

MEDITATION

Paradise Gardens
Geoff Hamilton (BBC Books,
1997)

Teach Yourself to Meditate
Eric Harrison (Piatkus, 1994)

How to Relax
Mike George (Duncan Baird
Publishers, 1998)

Creating Japanese Gardens
Philip Cave (Aurum Press,
1993)

*A Japanese Touch for Your
Garden*
K M Seike and D H Engel
(Kodansha International,
1992)

Index

For Dean, the wind beneath my wings

Author's acknowledgements

I am eternally grateful to Susan Haynes at Weidenfeld & Nicolson for both her warm reception of my initial ideas and her faith in my ability to 'deliver the goods'; also to my editor, Maggie Ramsay, for her enduring good humour and her ability to make sense of my ramblings. I would also like to thank the remainder of the team at W&N for producing such a beautiful book.

A huge thank you to my agent, Charlotte Howard, for her enthusiasm and optimism right from the outset and for guiding me along what has been a very steep learning curve!

Many, many thanks to Will Ryan and Jen Winter for being so liberal with their red pens and particularly to Will for being such a terrific 'lay person'! I cannot even begin to put into words my gratitude to Jen for her sound advice and unwavering support.

I also owe a great deal to my professional proofreaders for their practical guidance; I have learnt so much from all of them:
Feng shui: Graham Gunn; Richard Creightmore
Colour therapy: Janet Wells
Herbalism: Jenny Jones
Aromatherapy: Juanita Freeth
Meditation: Bill Heilbronn (yoga); Robert Ketchell and Kira Dalton of the Japanese Garden Society

The author and publishers would like to thank Laurence Pollinger Ltd (London), Viking Penguin Inc. (New York) and the Estate of Frieda Lawrence Ravagli for permission to reproduce the extract on page 65 from 'Red Geranium and Godly Mignonette', from The Complete Poems of D H Lawrence. *Other sources: page 6, from* Gardens are for People *by Thomas D Church (Reinhold, New York, 1955); page 89, from* Twelve Healers and Other Remedies *by Edward Bach (C W Daniel, 1952) Every care has been taken to trace copyright owners, but if we have omitted anyone we apologize and will, if informed, make corrections in any future edition.*

Picture credits

JERRY HARPUR: 8 Coton Manor, Northamptonshire; 10 Designer: Gunilla Pickard, Great Waltham, Essex; 21 Charles Cresson, Philadelphia, USA; 32 Sticky Wicket, Buckland Newton, Dorset; 38 Designer: Ian Teh, London; 53 Coombelands, Pulborough, Sussex; 58–9 Designer: Greg Abramowitz, Los Angeles, USA; 63 Designer: Cyrille Schiff, Los Angeles, USA; 134 (bottom right) Iden Croft Herbs, Staplehurst, Kent; John Scarman, Staffordshire; 150 Designer: Gunilla Pickard, Great Waltham, Essex; 156–7 Designer: Gunilla Pickard, Great Waltham, Essex; 160–61 Ryoan-ji temple, Kyoto, Japan.
DEREK HARRIS: 22; 24; 45; 51; 54–5; 64; 68–9; 72–3; 129; 143; 148; 156 (left).
ANNE HYDE: 7.
CLIVE NICHOLS: 2 Roger Platts, Chelsea 97; 3; 4; 12 (bottom) Designer: Mark Brown; 19 The Anchorage, Kent; 25; 28 The Anchorage, Kent; 37 Graham Strong/Clive Nichols; 62 Designer: Jane and Clive Nichols; 74 Sticky Wicket, Dorset, Designer: Pam Lewis; 87 (left); 88 Le Manoir aux Quat'Saisons, Oxfordshire; 95 Tudor House, Southampton; 99 Designer: Julie Toll, Chelsea 94; 102-3 Barnsley House, Gloucestershire; 124 National Asthma Campaign, Chelsea 93; 134 (top right); 134 (bottom left); 147; 149.
SCIENCE PHOTO LIBRARY: 34; 159.
JUSTYN WILLSMORE: 12 (top) RHS Wisley; 14 Abbotsbury; 27 Sir Harold Hillier Gardens & Arboretum (HH); 30 Chenies Aquatics; 35 (top) HH; 35 (bottom) HH; 71 BBC Gardeners World; 77 (left) RHS Wisley; 77 (right) HH; 79 (left) HH; 79 (right) RHS Wisley; 81 (left) Mr & Mrs Willsmore; 81 (right) HH; 82 HH; 83 (left) HH; 83 (right) RHS Wisley; 85 (left) HH; 85 (right) Chelsea Physic Garden; 87 (right); 104 (left and right) RHS Wisley; 105 HH; 107 HH; 108 (left and right) HH; 109 RHS Wisley; 110 (top) HH; 110 (bottom); 111 HH; 112 RHS Wisley; 114 RHS Wisley; 115 RHS Wisley; 121 HH; 123 HH; 134 (top left) Wisley; 134 (centre) HH; 144 RHS Wisley; 145 HH; 163 The Sound of Water; 165; 166 HH; 167 (top) HH; 167 (bottom) HH.

First published in Great Britain in 1998
by George Weidenfeld & Nicolson

This paperback edition first published
in 1999 by
Seven Dials, Illustrated Division
The Orion Publishing Group
Wellington House, 125 Strand
London, WC2R 0BB

A CIP catalogue record for this book is available from the British Library.
ISBN 1 84188 033 7

Art Director: David Rowley
Editor: Maggie Ramsay
Designed by Nigel Soper
Illustrations by Ruth Lindsay

Set in Helvetica Neue and Sabon
Printed and bound in Italy